MICHAEL JENNER

Fit in 15 at 60+!

THE COMPLETE HOME WORKOUT FOR SENIORS

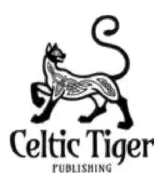

Celtic Tiger
PUBLISHING

Table of Contents

Introduction IX

Chapter 1: Fitness at Any Age...1

Common Myths 2

Myth: Loss of Energy in Advanced age is Inevitable—There is no Point! 2

Myth: Exercise is not Safe for People our age Because There is an Inherent Risk of Injury. 3

Myth: I Need to Check With my Doctor Before I Start to Exercise..................................3

Myth: I am Sick, so I Should not Exercise. OR I'm in Pain, so I Should not Exercise 4

Myth: I Have Never Exercised, so it is too Late to Make a Change to my Health. 5

Myth: I do not Have Time...5

Myth: I am too Weak to Start Exercising. 5

Myth: I am Disabled, so I Cannot Exercise 6

Myth: I Cannot Afford it 6

Myth: Exercise is Boring. 6

Myth: I Have Been Doing the Same Workout Program for Years and do not see why I Should Change 7

Myth: The Easiest Method to Avoid Falling is to Avoid Doing Anything........................7

Benefits of Exercising 7

Exercise Protects Against Chronic Diseases. 8

Exercise Boosts Immunity. 8

Exercise Prevents Bone Loss. 9

Maintaining Your Weight is Easier with Exercise 9

Exercise Improves Mental Health. 9

Exercise can Help You Sleep Better 10

Exercise Can Help You Feel Better If You Have Osteoarthritis. 10

Exercise Supports Healthy Social Interaction 11

Exercise Helps Keep Your Brain in Good Shape 11

Exercise Improves Cardiovascular Strength 11

Exercise Helps You Keep Your Independence. 12

Frequently Asked Questions About Exercising in Your 60s 12

How Long Should I Exercise Daily? 12

Which Exercises are Best for Older Adults? 12

How do I Stay Committed to Regular Physical Exercise? 13

Is it Safe for Seniors to Exercise? 14

How Often Should I Exercise? 14

Where Should I Start if I Have not Exercised in Years? 14

Do I Need to Consult a Doctor Before Starting a Physical Activity Program? 15

Do I Need a Particular Outfit or Equipment for Exercise? 15

Chapter 2: Breaking Down the Major Muscle Groups **17**

The Basics 18

Major Muscle Groups 18

Chest 19

Back 20

Arms 22

Shoulder 22

Abdominals 23

Legs 24

Chapter 3: The Importance of Stretching **27**

Why is Stretching Important? 28

Do I Need to Stretch Every Muscle? 28

What are the Benefits of Stretching? 28

How do I Stretch Correctly? 30

What Things I Should Avoid During Stretching? 31

What is the Best Time to Stretch? 31

Remember 31

Types of Stretching 32

    Static Stretching 32

    Dynamic Stretching... 33

Simple Stretches for You 33

    Neck Stretches.. 33

    Back Stretches 39

    Lower Body Stretches 43

    Upper Body Stretches 48

    Advanced Stretching Exercises 52

Chapter 4: Core Strength Is Critical............................57

What are the Core Muscles? 58

Why are Core Muscle Exercises Important? 59

    In the Office 61

    At Home 61

    Engaging in Hobbies 62

How do I Build a Strong Core? 62

    Exercises 62

Chapter 5: Strength Training is not Just for Gym Rats 65

Types of Strength Training 67

Benefits of Strength Training 69

Chapter 6: 21 Bodyweight Exercises in 21 days **73**

Make it a Habit 73

Step 1 74

Step 2 74

Step 3 75

The Routine 75

Week 1 76

Week 2 83

Week 3 90

Chapter 7: 21 Strength Training Moves **99**

21 Weighted Exercises 101

Chapter 8: Exercise Modifications: Obesity **123**

Warm-ups 124

Gastrocnemius Stretch 124

Gastrocnemius stretch sounds difficult but is very easy to do. 124

Exercises 127

Core Exercises 131

Low impact cardio 135

Weight training 135

Diet 135

Chapter 9: Exercise Modifications: Arthritis **137**

How Exercise Helps 137

Exercises for the Arthritis Patient 138

    Range of Motion Exercises 138

    Strengthening Exercises 139

    Aerobic Exercises 139

    Tips to Protect Your Joints 139

Chapter 10: Exercise Modifications: Bad Knees 141

Stretches 142

Strength 145

Tips 154

    Keep a Proper Body Weight 154

    Maintain a Regular Workout Schedule 155

    Steer Clear of Injuries 155

    Don't discount mobility and stretching 155

Chapter 11: Exercise Modifications: Heart Conditions 157

Preparation 158

Aerobic Exercises 159

    Jogging and Running 159

    Swimming 160

Strength Training 161

Flexibility 163

FAQs About Exercises After a Heart Attack or Surgery 163

Chapter 12: Making Exercise a Habit, not a Chore 167

Building a Balanced Exercise Plan 169

Tips for Staying Consistent 169

Conclusion 173

Introduction

"Age is not lost youth but a new stage of opportunity and strength"

Betty Friedan

Do you remember the last time you woke up with the sun and went for a run? What about the last time you went for a swim? By swimming, I don't mean just lounging in the water. No, I am talking about an actual swim— at least a few laps of the pool. It has been a while, hasn't it? For many of us, it has.

For most people, working out is not a daily habit. Sure, most of us have jogged or gone to the gym at some point in our lives. Yet, as we grew older, the habits discontinued, and there simply was no time or interest left for daily workouts. It was fine, until it wasn't. You don't really understand what lack of exercise will do to you until you are well into your 60s and suddenly, the chores you have been doing for the last 30 years seem daunting. A bit of gardening leaves you with sore knees and a stiff back, walking through the grocery store or shopping mall leaves you exhausted, and you can't even stand up suddenly without popping a few joints. As for getting out of bed in the morning...

If you are already someone who is going through this, you must be wondering why I am making you relive all that bad stuff. There is a point; I promise! So, here's the thing. Most people our age are going through exactly the same thing, and a majority of them actually believe there is nothing to be done. They think they have spent too many years not exercising and their joints are now too stiff and their muscles too weak. Others, to their credit, tried doing exercises and even going to the gym. However, after just a few weeks of trying to run on a fancy treadmill and one ankle sprain later, they have also given up.

At this point, there is only one question that matters: Is it, or is it not possible to gain back the mobility and the strength we have lost? In a word, YES! It is definitely possible, and it is possible without having to buy any expensive equipment, take out gym memberships, or get any surgery. All you need is a simple, methodical exercise regime that you can do by yourself from the comfort of your home. "Yes, yes," I hear you say, "that's all fine and good, but I have tried that, and it never worked for me." Trust me, you really can. How do I know? Because I have been through the same things! I have been a moderately active guy my whole life. I have walked, jogged, swam, and been a regular gym member. I even did manual labor back in the day. I tried to take up those habits again when I could feel myself getting weaker and older. I will tell you now, that was a big mistake. Taking my 60-year-old body to do the workouts designed for someone in their 30s or 40s only made me tired, miserable, and ready to give up. Then, I did the only thing that made sense. I researched, consulted physicians, asked personal trainers, and even went through a good number of journals (you will see them mentioned throughout the book) to create a customized exercise routine for my body and my age. Needless to say, it worked! I now enjoy more mobility, fewer aches and pain, and far greater strength than I have felt in ages.

During my research, I learned a lot about the human body, physiology, and the muscular system. Only then, did I find out why traditional exercises at the gym don't work for people like us. Our metabolism, muscles, and cellular turnover rates are quite different from the average adults. Everything is much slower. In fact, traditional heavy exercises can actually harm your body by the sudden increase of oxygen in the muscles (Ji, 2001)[1]. Unsurprisingly, a different approach is needed. The generic ones are not tailored to your body's needs nor based on your limits. You need to fix what is lacking in your exercise routine. In this book, I will teach you how.

This book is a one-stop solution to your mobility problems. No, relaxing on the couch won't magically solve all your health problems in 21 days, thats for sure. However, I will show you how to build back your energy and core strength little by little, day by day, without injuring yourself. Also, since I know you will probably have problems sticking to a routine, I have included some simple tips and tricks to ensure you don't skip exercises and actually enjoy them. To top it off, this book is largely based on scientific evidence and cited throughout; so, if you find something you want more information on, you can look it up.

So, you may be wondering who I am and why you should listen to me. A valid question. I won't pretend to be an expert with formal education in sports physiology. However, I do have one of the most important factors that perhaps no other writer or gym instructor can offer: I am in my 60s! I have gone through the same struggles and faced questions you are facing now. "Am I becoming too old?" "Will I be able live independently as time goes on?" "Will I need to move or hire someone to live with me?" These worries hounded me. Some things in life you just need to experience yourself to appreciate what it means—both physically and mentally. After a few years of trial and error, I finally managed to get to where I am comfortable and confident in my body. At our age, that is what matters.

That being said, nothing in this book is contradictory to current medical practices and mentions no medical treatment alternatives. Meaning, even though I will give you step-by-step instructions to a few exercises that will help you keep your sugar levels down, you still need to take insulin for your diabetes!

Moving into our 60s should be a sweet age. Some of us may be lucky and have retired, most of us will at least be starting to think about those retirement plans. Our children will have grown up, so we are left with no little kids 24/7 and perhaps no job to worry about. More importantly, we have more time to ourselves.

For many, it really is the best time, for others, not so much. For those struggling, as I have, this book is for you. Think of it as a gift from a friend who wants you to enjoy your remaining days in peace and health.

I would recommend that before you start any of the exercises, please read the book from cover to cover. That way, you will get the overall picture of what will bring you success without the risk of hurting yourself in the process. You will see that there is an entire chapter on the importance of incorporating stretching exercises into your daily routine, that will transform your fitness levels. I have also included an additional set of 21 exercises that use light weights and are a little more strenuous. These are an option once you have spent a few months getting back into shape. By all means, add them gradually as you start to feel those joints becoming more supple and those muscles more capable of work.

Now, go get fit!

Resources:

1. Ji, L. L. (2001). Exercise at old age: Does it increase or alleviate oxidative stress? Annals of the New York Academy of Sciences, 928(1), 236-247.

Chapter 1: Fitness at Any Age

"You are never too old, and it's never too late"
Michael Jenner

O ur progression in life is marked and measured with milestones that make us look forward to the future. Our first serious relationship, getting the job we always wanted, being promoted, buying our first house, or starting a family are only some of the goals that keep us going. Growing up has its advantages, such as the freedom to live your life on your own terms, the wisdom that comes with age, and the ability to spend more time with family and friends. Every year, we learn something new that broadens our horizons and aids our emotional and spiritual development. Perhaps the only disadvantage of growing older is losing energy to engage in physical activities such as running errands, cleaning the house or car, enjoying a rough and tumble with the grandchildren, or just walking the dog. Simple tasks that should be easy become harder with age. To make it worse, it's not even a smooth decline! One day, you are doing great; you are exercising and gaining more mobility. All of the sudden, after just one or two days of inactivity, you wake with pain and return to square one.

For me, this frustration felt even more acute during the COVID-19 pandemic. As most of us were stuck indoors, with no way of going out or getting simple exercises, it was indeed tough to keep strength and mobility in our bones. The first year was especially rough, wasn't it? There was no cure in sight. So, we were stuck indoors, with no way of exercising and a constantly worsening knee pain, backache, or whatever you were suffering from. The bottom line is, it was awful, it was sudden, it can happen again, and we need to find a solution.

Common Myths

Another consequence of inactivity, aside from chronic pain, can be the loss of freedom. For me, I remember getting to the point that I could not turn my head over my shoulder driving, which made joining the freeway dangerous! It is easy to lose our capacity to do the everyday routine things. These things that it seemed not so long ago we didn't even think about, and we just did them. While it's true that you can't expect to be as active in your 60s as you were in your 30s or 40s, routine exercise can do wonders for your overall physical health. If you are one of those people who believe they are too out of shape, ill, exhausted, or just plain unhealthy to exercise, I am here to explain why you're mistaken. This chapter will bust some common myths and misconceptions about exercise at old age and help you get one step closer to your optimal health level. It's all about being the best version of yourself.

Myth: Loss of Energy in Advanced age is Inevitable—There is no Point!

If this were true, we wouldn't see bodybuilders and marathon runners in their 70s, 80s, or even 90s excelling at their careers. This might come as a surprise, but energy loss comes from the lack of inactivity, not aging. Regular exercise helps you become stronger, reduces bone loss, boosts balance and coordination, enhances your mood, increases your memory, and can alleviate the symptoms of various chronic illnesses. Exercise benefits our health in more ways than one. It helps with memory and dementia prevention. It can also assist you in maintaining your independence and way of life. We'll keep doing the things we enjoy as we get older if we stay strong and flexible. You'll also be less likely to require assistance. We all want to maintain our independence for as long as we can!

Myth: Exercise is not Safe for People our age Because There is an Inherent Risk of Injury.

Even though this is a clear risk, we can take measures to improve balance and flexibility—particularly through exercise. Many people want to begin exercising, but they are terrified of falling or injuring themselves, no one wants a hip fracture right?. However, there is genuinely no reason to worry. I recommend that you take on balance and flexibility exercises first to ensure that you are capable and confident in your movements. Exercise, in fact, has been shown to lessen the risk of falling. Strength, balance, and agility are all improved by practice. Tai Chi and other balance-enhancing exercises may be particularly beneficial. Are you concerned about osteoporosis and brittle bones? Regular exercise is one of the most effective strategies to strengthen your bones.

Myth: I Need to Check With my Doctor Before I Start to Exercise

Exercising on a daily basis can help you lose weight, lower your risk of heart disease, and strengthen your bones and muscles. As long as you take it slow and do not overdo it, you should be fine. However, if it's been a long time since you've exercised and you have any health problems or issues, you should consult your doctor before beginning a new fitness plan.

Although most of us can safely engage in moderate physical activity, such as brisk walking, health experts advise that you consult your doctor before beginning an exercise program if any of the following apply:

- You have a cardiac condition.
- You have severe uncontrolled diabetes type 1 or type 2.
- You are suffering from kidney disease.
- You suffer from arthritis.
- You are undergoing cancer treatment or have recently completed cancer treatment.

- Your blood pressure is too high.

Suppose you haven't exercised consistently in a long time. In that case, you can generally begin by exercising at a mild to a moderate level and gradually increase your activity without visiting a doctor. After starting an exercise program, you should consult your doctor if you experience symptoms that could indicate a heart, lung, or other significant ailments, such as:

- You have pain or discomfort in your chest, neck, jaw, or arms at rest or during physical activity.
- Exercise or exertion causes dizziness, lightheadedness, or fainting.
- You experience shortness of breath during light exercise, at rest, when lying down, or getting ready for bed.
- You notice swelling of the ankles, especially at night.
- You have a heartbeat that is fast or pronounced (you can hear it).
- You have a cardiac murmur that has been previously diagnosed by your doctor.
- You experience vomiting or stomach upset after exercising.

Myth: I am Sick, so I Should not Exercise. OR I'm in Pain, so I Should not Exercise.

This is another outdated idea that has done us a great injustice! We already know that exercise is one of the most effective strategies to strengthen bones and protect joints. Our muscle mass increases, the blood supply increases, and not to mention the endorphins (happy hormones) that get released when you exercise. The overall effect is: you experience less pain! It aids osteoporosis patients in avoiding crippling fractures, controls blood sugar in the diabetic, and reduces cholesterol in heart block patients. Exercise is almost always a good suggestion if you have a chronic health concern. Consult your doctor first, but exercise will almost certainly help.

Myth: I Have Never Exercised, so it is too Late to Make a Change to my Health.

It's true that engaging in physical activity throughout our lives increases our chances of being healthy as we age. However, experts assure us that individuals who have led an inactive lifestyle can benefit from starting a regular exercise regimen at any age—whether they are 60, 70, 80, or older. For example, beginning an exercise practice can enhance muscle strength even in adults in their nineties who live in nursing homes, according to studies. In addition, other evidence suggests that beginning exercise late in life can reduce the likelihood of developing health problems, such as diabetes, and improve symptom management.

Myth: I do not Have Time.

This is a frequent misconception among people of all ages. A minimum of 120 minutes of aerobic exercise per week is recommended by experts. That seem like a lot. However, it only takes a little more than 15 minutes per day. Furthermore, you are not required to complete it all at once. It's possible to divide it up. Do some stretches for 5 minutes when you first get up. Take a 10-minute stroll in the morning and 5-10 minutes on a stationary bike in the evening, and you're done for the day. The important thing here is to build the healthy habit into your daily routine.

Myth: I am too Weak to Start Exercising.

The first step is always the most difficult. The good news is, there's a suitable exercise for people of all ages. Perhaps you've recently recovered from an illness or surgery and are unable to even walk around the block. Presumably, you only get out of your chair to use the restroom during the day. If that's the case, start from there! Decide to get out of your chair ten times today. Your strength will improve as you perform more, and you will be able to set higher goals.

Myth: I am Disabled, so I Cannot Exercise.

Although a disability can make things difficult, there is no reason you cannot exercise. For example, if you're in a wheelchair, you may get an aerobic workout and improve strength by using your arms. Even bedridden patients may find methods to exercise. Consult a doctor or physical therapist to see if any workouts may be modified to accommodate your impairment.

Myth: I Cannot Afford it.

Exercise doesn't always mean fancy equipment and complex body movements. We know that memberships to gyms and treadmills for home use can be costly. Still, that's no excuse for not working out. It is possible to work out for free. It costs nothing to go for a walk. Check out your local senior center for free demonstration classes. Soup cans or milk jugs loaded with sand can be used to hoist weights at home. Exercises to increase balance and flexibility can be done in your dining room chair. If you have a medical condition, your insurance may cover a few physical therapy or occupational therapy sessions. There are numerous low-cost or no-cost alternatives to get in shape.

Myth: Exercise is Boring.

You're not exercising properly if it's dull. Honestly, it doesn't even have to feel like you're exercising. Keep in mind that any form of physical activity counts. Physical activity can be anything from catching up with a friend while walking the mall, to taking a dance class, playing with your grandchildren, bowling, gardening, or volunteering with your local school system or park. Anything that causes your body to stay active can be counted as physical activity.

Myth: I Have Been Doing the Same Workout Program for Years and do not see why I Should Change.

First of all, well done on your hard work over the years! Yes, this may be a case of "if it ain't broke, don't fix it." On the other hand, our fitness requirements may fluctuate as we get older, and our health circumstances change. Certain exercises may no longer be safe, necessitating the use of low-impact, lower-intensity, or otherwise modified exercise. We may find that we are not covering all of the bases in terms of a thorough fitness regimen. This book will help you do just that.

Myth: The Easiest Method to Avoid Falling is to Avoid Doing Anything.

Unfortunately, that is not how it works. If you are averse to activity, you might save yourself from injuries, but your body will develop atrophies. Moreover, inactivity increases the danger of falling. This is how the cycle works:

1. You have a fall.

2. You reduce your level of activity because you are afraid of falling.

3. This depletes your energy reserves, muscular tone, and attentiveness, making it more likely that you may trip and fall again.

Ask your healthcare practitioner about a fall prevention exercise regimen that's perfect for you to avoid this deadly loop. If you use a cane, walker, or other mobility devices, be sure it's properly fitted and that you know how to use it.

Benefits of Exercising

Now that we have cleared up whatever misconceptions you might have regarding exercise, let's dive deeper into the rewards of exercising. We've been told that exercise is healthy for our hearts for a long time, but studies show that's only the beginning! Physical decline is slowed by maintaining an active lifestyle. Our lungs, muscles, bones, and joints are all protected by it. It lowers stress levels and strengthens our immune system. Many common health diseases, including arthritis, diabetes, stroke, renal disease, and depression, can be delayed or managed with exercise. It aids in the maintenance of a healthy weight and even lowers the risk of some malignancies. Exercise can help you fight the cognitive loss that comes with getting older, and many people are unaware that exercise can also aid in treating depression. According to studies, exercising builds brain connections and reduces the impact of stress and anxiety.

Exercise Protects Against Chronic Diseases.

Exercise protects against a variety of chronic diseases, including cardiovascular disease, colon cancer, diabetes, obesity, and hypertension. In addition, physical activity can help you manage symptoms if you already have a chronic illness. It may even aid in the prevention of cognitive deterioration. For example, according to one study, participants over the age of 60 were shown to have fewer Alzheimer's disease biomarkers when they exercised for at least 15 minutes a day.

Regular physical activity has been demonstrated in studies to help prevent a variety of ailments, including heart disease and diabetes. Physical activity that emphasizes aerobic workouts is beneficial to the heart, blood vessels, and lungs since it enhances breathing and heart rate. You can delay or lessen your chance of some diseases, including breast, colon, and lung cancer, as well as diabetes and heart disease, by keeping these essential organs healthy.

Exercise Boosts Immunity.

Exercise boosts overall immune function, which is especially crucial for us seniors whose immune systems are frequently weakened. Even light activity, such as walking, can be an effective aid in the management of avoidable diseases. Moderate exercise was linked to a lower incidence of acute respiratory disease and fewer sick days in a 2018 study. The exact mechanism through which exercise boosts immunity is unknown. There are, however, numerous theories. Some scientists believe that physical activity's anti-inflammatory properties help the immune system work better. Immune cells' performance may also be improved by exercise.

Exercise Prevents Bone Loss.

As we become older, both men and women lose bone density, with postmenopausal women losing up to 2% every year. Muscle toning has been demonstrated to slow the loss of bone density and even repair it. Stronger bones reduce the risk of fractures and can also help with balance. Exercise can help seniors live independently for longer by reducing the risk of falls and injuries. In addition, the body gradually weakens as we age, leading to a loss of freedom. You may strengthen your muscles and enhance your flexibility, balance, and coordination by engaging in regular physical activity. As a result, you'll be less likely to fall and will be able to preserve your mobility and freedom.

Maintaining Your Weight is Easier with Exercise.

With age, metabolism slows, producing weight gain and making it more challenging to maintain a healthy weight. Regular exercise can help you burn more calories and lose weight by increasing your metabolism and strengthening your muscles. Inactive bodies tend to gain weight that gets increasingly difficult to shred as we age. Obesity comes with a whole set of health complexities, which is why it's essential to stay active regularly.

Exercise Improves Mental Health.

Exercising has a multitude of mental health benefits. It can aid in the relief of anxiety and depression symptoms, as well as promote relaxation and a general sense of well-being. A 2019 study of adult men aged 65 and up discovered that the mood-boosting effects of exercise last far into old age—which is why staying active is so important. Us seniors benefit because exercise releases endorphins into the brain and reduces despair. As a result, your mood will improve. According to Michael Otto, Ph.D., a psychology professor at Boston University, physical fitness can improve one's mood relatively quickly, as per the American Psychological Association. "There's a really substantial correlation between exercise and mood," he stated. "Mood enhancement usually occurs within five minutes of moderate activity." Exercising isn't just a stress reliever. Your confidence is likely to rise when you begin to experience outcomes from exercising over time. It's natural to suffer depression as we get older, whether it's due to shifting schedules or a sense of loss of purpose after retiring and no longer working. Exercising causes your body to release natural chemicals which brightens your mood and makes you feel happy. This is a better alternative to over-the-counter medication.

Exercise can Help You Sleep Better.

Do you have trouble falling asleep at night on a regular basis? Don't take sleeping pills; instead, start exercising! Because of the variations in body temperature before and after a workout, regular exercise can help us fall asleep faster. It also aids in the induction of deeper sleep, allowing you to wake up feeling refreshed and energized. This component of exercise is beneficial to us seniors because our bodies slow down as we age. In addition, a night of good sleep can assist in maintaining optimal cognitive and physical functioning (such as concentration, standard movements, and memory) throughout the day, lowering the chance of injury.

Exercise Can Help You Feel Better If You Have Osteoarthritis.

While it may seem contradictory, moving more can actually aid in the reduction of arthritic pain and stiffness. Low-impact aerobic activity, strength training, and range-of-motion exercises are all examples of arthritis-friendly exercises. What role does exercise play in the treatment of arthritis? It relieves pressure on hurting joints by strengthening the muscles around them. Physical activity can also assist in relieving pain and stiffness by reducing joint inflammation and increasing lubrication.

Exercise Supports Healthy Social Interaction.

Exercise can be turned into an enjoyable social event by joining a walking group, attending group fitness courses, or visiting a gardening club. This forces folks to retain a sense of purpose and avoid feelings of loneliness or sadness. These exercise-based social groups help maintain strong social links. Above all, choose an activity that you enjoy, and it will never feel like a big deal again.

Exercise Helps Keep Your Brain in Good Shape.

Exercise not only strengthens your bones and muscles, but it also benefits your mind! You're being inventive and multitasking, no matter how you choose to exercise, keeping the brain happy and engaged. This can help to prevent memory loss and cognitive decline, as well as minimize the risk of dementia.

Exercise Improves Cardiovascular Strength.

Regardless of whether you choose cardio (like jogging and swimming) or strength training (like lifting and resistance), exercise benefits us seniors by increasing our endurance. As a result, simple activities like climbing stairs, doing domestic tasks, or engaging in your favorite hobbies will be simple to maintain as you age. "Incorporating exercise into your daily routine will drastically enhance your cardiovascular performance by boosting your heart and lowering overall blood pressure, resulting in increased endurance and energy levels," says one study.

Exercise Helps You Keep Your Independence.

This is possibly the most crucial advantage of exercising as you get older. While care homes are necessary for some, many would like to remain in their own homes for as long as possible. Therefore, it's critical to stick to a workout routine that promotes this way of life.

Frequently Asked Questions About Exercising in Your 60s

How Long Should I Exercise Daily?

Aim for at least 100-120 minutes of medium-intensity aerobic activity each week, as well as two days of weight training per week when you get to that stage. However, begin by doing what you can and progressively expand your efforts. It is ok to take it in stages and start slowly, especially if you haven't been active in a while. After a few weeks or months, increase the duration and frequency of your activities. As I have mentioned already, make this a daily habit. It can take a while, and evidence suggests that a new habit takes just 66 days to become automatic.

Which Exercises are Best for Older Adults?

An older adult's fitness plan should include aerobic activity, strength/resistance training, and stretching/flexibility activities. Trendy fitness programs and high-intensity workouts aren't viable or safe options for most of us senior folks. Below, are some excellent training options that can help you increase your agility, stamina, balance, and coordination.

- **Yoga is a low-impact activity that is gentle on the joints.** At the same time, it aids in the development of muscles, the stabilization of your core, the improvement of flexibility, and the strengthening of your bones.

To help you grasp basic positions, look for a beginning yoga session in your region. Some yoga programs are tailored to the needs of senior citizens and incorporate both seated and standing poses.

- **Pilates, like yoga, provides a good workout while being easy on the joints.** It focuses on strengthening the core to enhance balance and stability, and it has been demonstrated to alleviate the symptoms of arthritis, MS, and Parkinson's disease. Many of the workouts are done while sitting or lying down. If you haven't exercised in a long time, Pilates is an excellent alternative to explore.

- **Aerobic exercises help build endurance.** Including an aerobic endurance activity in your day will help you increase your overall stamina, strengthen your lungs and airways, and improve your cardiovascular function. What is aerobic exercise? Walking, swimming, and riding a stationary bike are all viable options for us older folks. The suggested amount of time is thirty minutes every day. This can be broken up into three 10-minute periods throughout the day.

- **Strength training has many benefits.** No, we're not referring to bench pressing a hundred pounds here! You may reverse muscle loss and burn body fat at home by using basic, low-impact bodyweight training activities. Wall pushups, stair climbing, squats, and single-leg stands are among them. Light hand weights (1 to 2 lbs) or resistance bands are also used in strength-training exercises. Aim for two to three times per week to get the most out of your workouts.

How do I Stay Committed to Regular Physical Exercise?

If you find it hard to stay motivated to exercise every day, find yourself a partner. It's sometimes more fun to exercise with a companion. If you don't have a workout partner, a community-based program might provide the social connection and encouragement you need to stick with it. Exercising in a social setting also adds a degree of safety for older persons who require additional supervision while doing physical activities.

Is it Safe for Seniors to Exercise?

Even those with chronic diseases and mobility issues can exercise safely once they reach the age of 60+. However, before beginning any exercise program, speak with your doctor to determine which options and degree of activity are best for your health. Then, you'll be able to discover firsthand the numerous and well-documented advantages of exercise.

How Often Should I Exercise?

Physical activity should be spaced out throughout the week, with a goal of being active at least 3-5 days each week. You might be able to find a method to be active every day of the week if you choose activities that you enjoy, are convenient, and economical. Make an effort to vary your activity routine so that you aren't doing the same thing every day. On some days, you might go for a stroll with a friend or family member in your neighborhood, while on others, you might participate in a more scheduled exercise program at a senior center or church. Many people discover that wearing a step counter assists them in keeping track of their activities.

Where Should I Start if I Have not Exercised in Years?

Give up on the old adage "no pain, no gain" because it's just not true! Too many of us were taught as children that physical activity must be painful or demanding in order to be beneficial. There are numerous wonderful solutions for those of us who are unable to exercise hard. Walking is a practical idea to boost your physical activity. Stretching, Tai Chi, and water exercise are all excellent choices. Gardening and working outside can also be beneficial forms of exercise and of course, following the exercises in this book is also a great start. Keep in mind that the most essential thing is not what you do but rather that you avoid immobility.

Do I Need to Consult a Doctor Before Starting a Physical Activity Program?

Seeing your doctor on a regular basis is always a good idea. In an ideal world, everyone would consult their doctor before making any changes to their exercise level. Unfortunately, many of us older folk are unable to see our doctors. The vast majority of us seniors can safely. Therefore, inactivity and sedentary living should not be excused since you don't have a doctor. The vast majority of older persons can safely discover an activity program that is both safe and productive for them. If you don't have a doctor, an exercise specialist or other health professionals may be able to help you. In most locations, a gym, YMCA, or health club can give you guidance regarding the appropriate exercise for you.

Do I Need a Particular Outfit or Equipment for Exercise?

No, thank you! It is unlikely that special attire or equipment is necessary to exercise. Wearing comfortable street shoes and ordinary loose-fitting clothes is sufficient for safe and effective physical activity. Cheap equipment, such as elastic bands and water-filled jugs, can be used to perform effective strength training. Online stores such as Amazon have a huge choice of cost-effective light weights and resistance bands.

Now that you know exercising is a healthy way of enriching your life, it should be easy to add it to your daily routine. Providing maximum movement and activity to your life, even in tiny amounts, can have a positive impact. It's never too late to get your body moving, improve your health and outlook, and improve how well you age, regardless of your age or physical condition.

The exercises in this book are designed to be accessible to the beginner, so even if you think you can't exercise, you'll find it easier than ever to get started. Far too often, we rely on excuses like "I'm too weak" or "I'm too out of shape," when we really need to be focusing on what we can be doing to improve our health. In the next chapter, we'll explore the major muscle groups that you work with when exercising. I have found that by understanding the functions served by each muscle, it is much easier to get into an exercising mindset. After all, you want to actually see the muscles you are working out, don't you?

*As with any other activity, it's essential that you listen to your body. As you go through the exercises in this book, remember to start slowly and focus on form. If you feel pain or discomfort, stop immediately and consult yourdoctor.

Chapter 2: Breaking Down the Major Muscle Groups

When I first started exercising, I didn't know much. All I had going for me was a need to change my life and my body for the better. So, I started with the traditional method that everyone follows. I started running, tried doing jumping jacks, and even tried to do some yoga. Suffice it to say, my exercise plan failed miserably. I saw no improvement, my pain was worse, and I even developed some new pains in my shoulders. It was a mess, and I honestly thought about giving up.

Then, another thought struck me. I was going about this the wrong way! I was exercising without having any knowledge about my body or the muscles I wanted to strengthen. This meant I was going into the exercise routines completely blind. I had no idea what muscles of my body were hurting or which ones I wanted to work on. My approach was not methodical, hence my results were not satisfactory.

Once I realized this, it was easy to see the gaps in my exercise routines. For example, I was suffering from shoulder pains, but I was running, which did nothing for my shoulders. Doing crunches didn't help my ankles either! I know you must be laughing at me right now but think about it! Most of us have been doing the same thing! By exercising and getting into shape, common folks just assume that it means running and swimming. We don't even consider what problems we want to solve. For some reason, it is generally assumed that whole-body exercises are supposed to help you solve most, if not all, muscle-related issues. The truth is, however, that just as different muscle groups work in different directions, their exercises are different too. As someone who wanted to regain strength and balance, it was very important for me to know about the individual muscle groups and how they interact.

The Basics

Let's start with the basics. What are the muscles? Well, muscles are groups of fibers or long threads of proteins. These protein fibers have the ability to stretch and contract on command. As they contract and expand, they control the movements of bones and organs. As you can imagine, not all muscles are the same. Some need to be controlled consciously, some need to be automated. Depending on the size and function, muscles can be of three types: smooth, skeletal, and cardiac. Smooth muscles line your internal organs and vessels, cardiac muscles form the heart and pump blood throughout the body, skeletal muscles control bones and body movement. Of these three muscle types, the first two are involuntary; hence, we will be primarily working with skeletal muscle.

Major Muscle Groups

Strictly speaking, there are many muscle groups that work individually and often along with other muscle groups. Their interactions are pretty complex. For example, the simple movement of moving your forearm requires several groups of muscles: one group to pull it into the desired direction, one to provide necessary resistance, one to hold the elbow steady, and one to hold the other muscles steady.

Broadly, for the sake of easy categorization and understanding, the skeletal muscles of the body can be divided into six major muscle groups. These, then, can be broken down into more specific sub-categories. The muscle groups are:

- Chest
- Back
- Arms
- Abdominals
- Legs
- Shoulders

Chest

Muscles of the chest cover the front side of your ribcage. As they cover your lungs and heart, these are important. The most prominent muscles of the chest are the pectoralis muscles. These give strength to your upper body and arms.

- **Pectoralis Major**: These muscles start from the middle bone of the chest and go sideways until they meet the upper arm bone. Basically, they cover more than 2/3 of the front of the chest. In a man, they are the large triangular-shaped muscles you see on the upper part of the chest. They are often referred to as the pectorals or "pecs." These muscles are the frontal connection of the arms to the chest. As you lift things with your arms or when you rotate your arms forward, these muscles are at work.

- **Pectoralis Minor:** These muscles lie beneath the pectoralis major and cover the rest of the front of the chest. They fall below and slightly anterior to the armpits. This set of muscles works in stabilization, rotation, and downward and forward movement of the scapula (shoulder blade). They also help in deep breathing by moving the ribs.

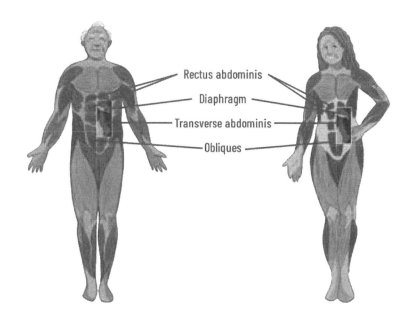

Rectus abdominis
Diaphragm
Transverse abdominis
Obliques

Back

The back is composed of five muscle groups:

- **Latissimus Dorsi (aka "lats"):** The latissimus dorsi are large, flat muscles that stretch to the sides, starting from the lower midline of the back, these muscles are trapezoidal. They are the broadest muscles of the back and cover almost all the lower and middle half of the back. Though situated in the lower and middle back, they control the movement of the upper part of the body, including movements of the arms and shoulders. If you have pain in the spine or shoulder, often it is due to these muscles.

- **Rhomboids:** Located in the upper back, rhomboids start from the midline and attach the scapula (shoulder bone) to the spine. So, they are holding the scapula in place. As the name implies, these muscles are rhomboidal in shape. You can't really see them as they lie beneath another muscle. Nevertheless, they are essential to strengthening the movements of the arm and shoulders.

- **Trapezius (aka "traps"):** The trapezius muscles cover the back of the neck and the upper part of the back. These muscles control the scapulae/shoulder blades and are involved in shrugging and neck movements. Most people, especially those who have desk jobs like me, have pain in the trapezius. You will feel the pain in the back and the upper portion of the shoulders and also where the neck and shoulders meet. They are used to tilt and turn the head and neck and provide support when you lift items over your head. Trapezius muscles also hold your posture.

- **Teres muscle:** These are small muscles on the back, close to the armpits. Found underneath the lats, the teres muscles help the upper arm in backward movements. They also hold the upper arm bone or humerus in place.

- **Erector spinae:** These are long strips of muscles. The erector spinae muscles lie on each side of the spine and go from the top (cervical vertebrae) to the bottom (lumbar vertebrae). True to their names, they help keep the spine "erect" and control side-to-side movements, as well as bending forward and sideways. Pain in the erector spinae is felt along the spine, along with a difficulty in standing straight or back spasms.

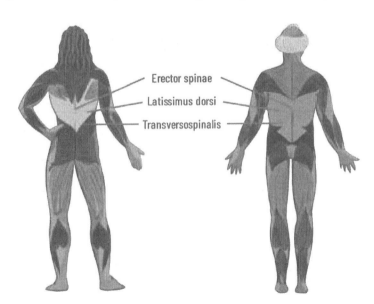

Arms

- **Biceps:** Biceps are the fleshy parts found in the front of the upper arm that gym rats like to show off. These muscles are the ones that flex the elbow. So, you need them for pretty much any heavy or moderate lifting you do. The bicep muscles give strength to the elbow, which is critical for lifting, and the shoulder. They help bend/curl the arm toward your body and assist in an upward movement of the shoulder.

- **Triceps:** Triceps are present in the lower or back surface of the upper arm. These muscles get very little attention, but are equally as crucial as the biceps as they help in arm extension. So, the movements you do while having the arm extended (washing the dishes or sweeping, for example) you are relying heavily on the triceps and the shoulder muscles. They also assist in stabilizing the shoulder joint. Triceps make the arm straight while the biceps pull it close or bend it. Both muscles are involved with fine motor movements like writing, drawing, pushing, and pulling, etc.

Shoulder

- **Deltoids (aka "delts"):** Known as the shoulder muscles, they provide support when you carry things and are used in all lifting motions. You will see that many exercises are focused on deltoids, along with the biceps, as they serve aesthetic purposes (making one look buff). You are unlikely to get any chronic pain here. However, it is not entirely useless, as you need a strong arm to lift your grandkids!

- **Rotator cuff:** These assist in the outward movement of the arm, flexing the arm, and lifting things.

Abdominals

Much of our upper body strength comes from the abdomen. Abdominal muscles are also responsible for good posture and flexibility. Unfortunately, these are also the muscles that get ignored the most. Even the healthiest people can have a lax abdomen and a belly pooch. While I am not saying, you need to get rid of that belly fat altogether and get a six-pack, if you want to be fit, you will at least need to strengthen a few key muscles in this area.

- **External Obliques:** These muscles line the sides of the abdomen. They help in keeping the shape of the abdominal cavity and aid the contraction of the diaphragm and chest. The obliques pull your chest down and make the chest cavity larger during a large intake of breath. They rotate the trunk on the same side (a side bend) or opposite sides (rotation). You may feel a sharp pain in this muscle when trying to rotate your body too fast or while reaching for something in the backseat. Obliques also help support the spine from the front and keep the intraabdominal pressure steady.

- **Serratus Anterior:** Sometimes referred to as "boxer's muscles." These muscles are placed just below and anterior to the armpits, lining the chest wall from the side and back. These are connected to the rib cage, which helps stabilize the shoulder and lift the ribs in a deep breath. They are responsible for the movement of the shoulder when you are pushing something or, although unlikely, throwing a punch. If you have a problem within this muscle, you will feel pain every time you try to push open a door or try to hang a towel, etc.

- **Psoas Major:** These muscles connect the upper and lower body. They are a major control point for hip joint flexion/movement. The psoas muscles also connect the inside of the skeleton to the outside and the upper back to the lower front. As you can imagine, in all sorts of twisting movements, the role of psoas muscles is extremely important. As they control much of hip joint movement, you are using them almost constantly during the day. When you are walking, standing, running, or even sitting, they are at work.

Legs

- **Hamstrings**: This huge muscle group is located in the upper back part of your thighs. They are responsible for most leg functions. Their primary function is to bend and extend your knees and propel your body forward when walking, running, or jumping. Even when you are standing up from a sitting position, you are using your "hams." If you have weak hams, you may find it difficult to stand up or lift your legs.

- **Quadriceps**: Also called "Quads," these are the second-largest major muscular group after the back and are located in the upper front of the thigh. This group consists of four muscles. They provide much of the strength of the knee. All of these muscles extend the leg and are responsible for extending the knee forward and upward. You need "quads" to go up the stairs or to get up from a chair and walk.

- **Gastrocnemius:** The calves are located in the back of the lower part of your legs. They move your lower legs and feet. Calve muscles are also very important for balance. They help in stabilizing your knee when you are putting your weight on a leg. Calves lock the knee in position—something many people struggle with. These muscles are essential for lifting your heels up and forward when walking, running, going upstairs, etc.

- **Gluteus Maximus:** Also named "glutes," are yet another muscle group that Instagrammers like. However, these are also crucial in balancing while standing. The gluteus maximus muscles attach to several places in the pelvis and thigh, allowing you to extend your upper leg, spread it, and turn it outward.

- **Gluteus Medius:** These connect the ilium (most prominent and uppermost bone of the hip) to the top of the femur (upper leg bone/thigh bone). The gluteus medius controls the movement of the hips and thighs. They also control the outward movement of the thighs, especially when you are putting weight on one leg. So, these muscles help in body balance. Those who had hip replacements or have had terrible falls oftentimes find it hard to regain strength in this muscle.

The muscles I described are hardly the only ones in your body. However, they are the most important ones for mobility and function, two things in which we are interested. So, we will focus mainly on these muscles in our exercise. After reading this chapter, try to identify these muscles in your body; get familiar with them. It is entirely okay if you can't find them all, but you will be, at the very least, able to identify the ones that are giving you grief! That is all you need to focus on exercising and strengthening these muscles!

Chapter 3: The Importance of Stretching

> *"Whatever kind of workout you settle on, it should include the Big Three of exercise for health and fitness. Aerobics, resistance exercises, and stretching!"*
>
> Jane Fonda

Now that you've learned about the muscle groups, I am sure you're anxious to try out a few moves but hold your horses! There is something you need to learn before you can do even the most basic exercise—warming up! Warming up before exercising is vital since you don't want to strain your muscles. There is a need to worry! Warming up does not include doing squats, jumping jacks, or anything else strenuous. It's simpler than that. We're talking about a crucial phase that you shouldn't overlook when getting ready to exercise—stretching. Muscle development and aerobic endurance are both essential for enhancing energy, balance, and speed. However, flexibility is another crucial part of health, which is where stretching comes in. Contrary to popular belief, gymnasts and yoga practitioners aren't the only ones who stretch. In order to get the maximum benefits, it must be a part of your daily routine.

Why is Stretching Important?

Stretching prevents sudden, excessive force from being applied to the muscles, which is important for maintaining the joints' range of motion. Muscles shorten and become tight due to lack of movement. As a result, when those muscles are called into action, they are feeble and unable to fully expand. You are very likely to suffer damage or even tear a few muscle fibers or ligaments if you were to suddenly start exercising with unstretched muscles.

Our muscle fibers are like elastic bands. With inactivity, they become less elastic. Sitting on the sofa all day, for example, causes tight hamstrings in the back of the leg. This can make it difficult to fully extend your leg or straighten your knee, preventing you from walking. Similarly, when tight muscles are abruptly called upon for a rigorous activity that strains them, such as tennis, they may be harmed as a result of the fast stretching. Muscles that have been injured may not be strong enough to support the joints, resulting in joint damage. Proper and regular stretching keeps muscles long, slender, and flexible. This means exercise "won't put excessive tension on the muscle tissue," according to Nolan, a physical therapist at Massachusetts General Hospital, which is associated with Harvard.

Do I Need to Stretch Every Muscle?

Nope, only the ones you want to work out with! You may be concerned that you must target each of the muscle groups you've just heard about, but don't be. You can target certain muscle groups to help you gain complete body flexibility. This chapter will show you how to incorporate key stretches into your daily practice.

What are the Benefits of Stretching?

- Stretching on a regular basis can help enhance your flexibility, which is vital for your general health. Improved flexibility can help you not only accomplish everyday tasks more efficiently, but it also helps postpone the loss of movement that comes with aging.

- Regular stretching might help you enhance your range of motion. You have more mobility when you can move a joint across its full range of motion.

- Dynamic stretches before physical activities have been found to help muscles prepare for that activity. They may also aid in the improvement of your sports or workout performance.

- Stretching on a regular basis may serve to strengthen circulation. Improved circulation enhances blood flow to your muscles, which can lessen muscular discomfort and speed up recovery time.

- Muscle imbalances are widespread, and they can result in bad posture. A combination of tightening and extending specific muscle groups helps alleviate joint pain and promote appropriate alignment, according to one study. This, in turn, may aid in the development of your posture.

- Your range of motion may be reduced as a result of tight muscles. When this happens, you increase your chances of hurting your back muscles. Stretching the muscles can aid in the healing of an existing back issue.

- There's a good probability your muscles are tense while you're under stress. This happens because your muscles tighten up in response to physical and emotional stress. Concentrate on your neck, shoulders, and upper back, as these are the parts of your body where you tend to keep your stress.

- Stretching daily will not only help you become more flexible, but it can also help you relax. Engage in mindfulness and meditation techniques while stretching to give your head a mental break.

- Tension and anxiety can cause headaches that make it challenging to go about your regular routine. Stretching, in addition to a healthy diet, appropriate hydration, and plenty of rest, can help relieve and prevent headache tension.

How do I Stretch Correctly?

Before you try stretching, make sure you're doing it correctly and safely. While stretching can be done at any time and in any location, the appropriate technique is essential. Stretching incorrectly might be bad for health. To make stretching safe, follow these guidelines:

Don't think of stretching as a warm-up. If you strain cold muscles, you risk injuring yourself. Warm-up for five to ten minutes with low-intensity walking, jogging, or biking before stretching. Stretching after an exercise, when your muscles are warm, is even better.

Make an effort to achieve symmetry. Flexibility is a hereditary trait that differs from person to person. Instead of aiming for the flexibility of a dancer or gymnast, concentrate on having equal flexibility on all sides of your body (especially if you have a history of previous injury). Flexibility that isn't equal on both sides could put you at risk of hurting yourself.

Concentrate on the primary muscle groups. Stretch your calves, thighs, waist, lower back, neck, and shoulders, among other important muscle groups. Make sure you extend all sides of your body. Also, stretch the muscles and joints that you utilize on a regular basis.

Make sure you don't bounce. Stretch in a smooth, non-bouncing motion. Bouncing when stretching can cause muscle injury and add to muscle tension.

Maintain your stretch. Breathe normally and hold each stretch for around 30 seconds; in troubled areas, hold for up to 60 seconds. While stretching, you should expect to experience tension rather than pain. You've gone too far if it aches. Hold the stretch once you've backed off to the point where you don't feel any pain.

Maintain your routine. Stretching can take a long time. Stretching frequently, at least two to three times a week, will provide the most benefits. If you don't stretch on a regular basis, you risk losing out on the possible benefits. If stretching helps you expand your range of motion, it's likely that if you stop stretching, your range of motion will diminish.

Incorporate movement into stretching. Gentle motions like Tai Chi and yoga might help you become more flexible with certain movements. These types of workouts can also help elderly folks avoid falling.

What Things I Should Avoid During Stretching?

Stretching is important, no doubt, but don't overdo it! One of the most important things to remember is to never extend a muscle that has been injured. Depending on the severity of the injury, you could wind up causing even more damage to the area and/or delaying tissue repair. You should always check with your doctor or physiotherapist before doing any exercise. This may sound obvious, but never push a stretch to the point of pain. It's OK to have a stretching sensation, but you should never undergo any pain.

What is the Best Time to Stretch?

The best time to perform these stretches for people who regularly exercise is at the start and the end of the activity, while your muscles are still warm and loose. A five-minute walk or jog before your workout is recommended.

However, stretching can be done at any time of day. It can be beneficial for people who are suffering from mobility loss. Even if you are not going to exercise immediately, stretching your muscles before bed or after waking up is a good way to get the blood pumping. You can even do some in the middle of the day or after you have been sitting for a while.

Remember

Before we get started, there are a few crucial reminders worth mentioning about stretching exercises.

1. **First and foremost, try to focus on your breathing during the stretches.** It's easy to overlook and not notice you're holding your breath when exercising. While it may seem easier or more convenient to hold your breath while stretching and exercising, the truth is that your muscles require oxygen to perform properly. So, take a deep breath and relax into each stretch, making sure not to hold your breath.

2. **Secondly, Do a warm up!** Warming up is required even before stretching. Many confuse between the two, but the warm-up procedure is done to increase blood flow to the muscles, while a stretching exercise lengthens the muscles fibers over and over so they are not rigid. Researchers also suggest at least a little warm up before all stretching. [1]

3. **Finally, never start a stretch cold and always take it slowly.** Before executing your stretches, make sure you warm up with some simple movements. Now that we've gone over the basics of stretching, it's time to look at the finest stretching exercises for seniors. Let's get this party started!

Types of Stretching

Static Stretching

Static stretching has been widely encouraged before engaging in physical exercise since the early 1980s as a way to avoid injury and improve physical performance. Muscles are flexed and held for a time frame in static stretches. The triceps stretch and the butterfly stretch are two examples of static stretches. Static stretching is a popular warm-up technique for exercise because it is thought that the slow, controlled movement allows the stretch to be performed easily and safely, with a lower risk of injury than other types of stretching. [2]

Dynamic Stretching

Active movements in which joints and muscles move through their complete range of motion are known as dynamic stretches. These can be used to help you warm up before you exercise. Dynamic stretches might be useful by simulating the movement of the activity or sport in which you're about to participate. A swimmer, for example, could circle their arms before entering the water. Dynamic stretches can also be a series of motions performed before any type of workout to get the body moving. Trunk twists, walking lunges, and leg swings against a wall are popular examples. [3]

Simple Stretches for You

Simple stretching exercises have been described below. Each of these exercises is to be carried out for 30 seconds, and special emphasis should be placed on ensuring that your breathing is normal throughout the activity. If you face difficulty stretching for 30 seconds, you can aim for 10-20 seconds and gradually work your way up.

Neck Stretches

Your neck never gets a break. It's always there, doing the crucial task of keeping your head up. Our technologically oriented ways haven't made things any easier. Stretching the neck helps to relieve tension in the areas that produce headaches and joint stiffness.

Flexion of the Neck:

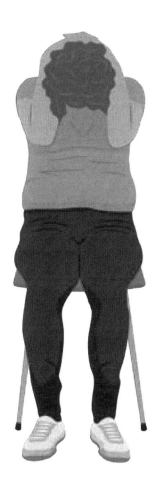

DIRECTIONS

1. Sit up straight in your chair, shoulders back and down.

2. Bring your chin as close to your chest as you are comfortable with. A stretch will be felt in the back of your neck.

3. Place your hands on the back of your head and apply slight pressure to increase the stretch.

4. Hold for the specified amount of time.

Neck Extension Stretch

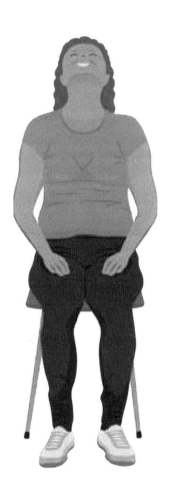

DIRECTIONS

1. Sit up straight in your chair, shoulders back and down.

2. Bring your head back as far as you can, staring up at the ceiling and as far as you feel comfortable. Do not push yourself to the point of pain.

3. Hold for a fixed amount of time, 10-30 seconds is fine, then gently bring your head back to center.

Neck Side Flexion Stretch

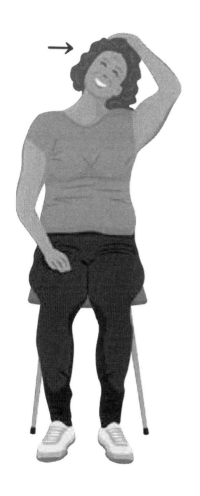

DIRECTIONS

1. Sit up straight in your chair, shoulders back and down.

2. Bring your ear to your shoulder's level. Keep your shoulder relaxed, and do not pull it up to your ear. Take it as far as you'd like.

3. Place your palm on the side of your head and apply slight pressure to improve the stretch.

4. Hold for the designated amount of time, say 30 seconds, and then switch sides.

Neck Rotation Stretch

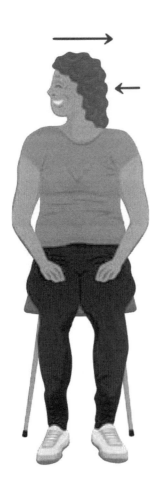

DIRECTIONS

1. Sit straight in your chair with your shoulders back and down.

2. Look to the side to the extent that you are comfortable.

3. Hold for 10-15 seconds then, switch sides.

Levator Scapulae Stretch

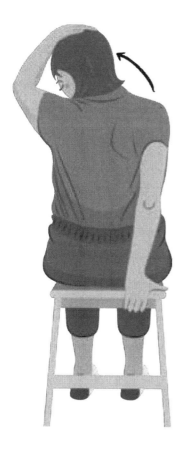

DIRECTIONS

1. Sit upright in your chair, shoulders back and down.

2. To stabilize your shoulder blade, place the hand of the side you're stretching behind the shoulder. If you are unable to do so, simply perform the exercise with one hand be- hind your shoulder.

3. Turn your head to one side at a 45-degree angle and lower your head as if you're staring at your knee on that side. When you glance behind the neck and shoulder on the opposite, you will feel a stretch. (This muscle is referred to as the Levator Scapular.)

4. Place your palm on the back of your head and apply slight pressure to increase the stretch.

5. Hold for the designated amount of time, then switch sides.

Back Stretches

Back stretching has several advantages, including reducing tension in the muscles that support the spine. As stress in these muscles can aggravate pain from a variety of back pain disorders, improving mobility in general with these stretches also lowers the likelihood of back pain-related impairment.

Lumbar Flexion Stretch

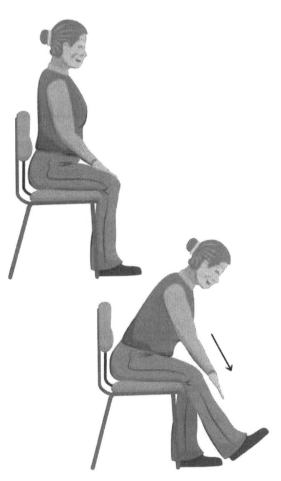

DIRECTIONS

1. Sit up straight in your chair, shoulders back and down.

2. Place your hands on your knees and your feet slightly out in front of you.

3. Slide your hands down your legs all the way to your feet, one at a time.

4. Hold for the specified amount of time before slowly sliding your hands back up.

Lumbar Side Stretch

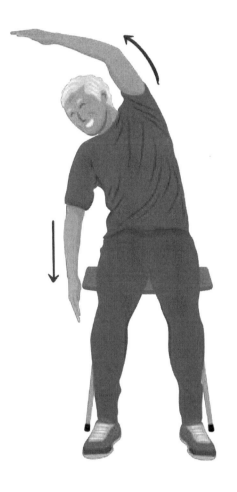

DIRECTIONS

1. Sit up straight in your chair, shoulders back and down.

2. One hand should be behind your head, and the other should be straight alongside you.

3. Slowly lower your straight arm to the side until you feel a stretch on the opposite side. (If placing your hand behind your head is difficult, keep it on your lap.)

4. Hold for the required amount of time, then switch sides.

Lumbar Extension Stretch

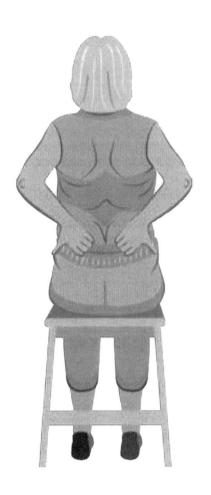

DIRECTIONS

1. To start, sit tall in the middle of your chair with your shoulders back and down.

2. Lean your lower back into your hands with your palms in the small of your back, feeling a stretch in your lower back. (Use the backs of your hands if you have trouble getting your palms around to the small of your back.)

3. Hold for a specified amount of time.

Rhomboids Stretch

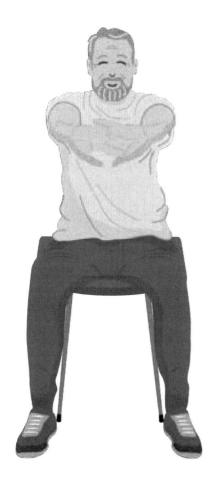

DIRECTIONS

1. Sit up straight in your chair, shoulders back and down.

2. Your fingers should be interlaced, and your palms should be facing away from you.

3. Bring your arms up to 90 degrees (or parallel to the floor) and push your hands out as far as you can while remaining upright. Your shoulder blades are stretching apart.

4. Return to the starting location after 10-30 seconds.

Lower Body Stretches

The standing quadriceps stretch is the first exercise on our list. It is an excellent stretching exercise for seniors since it is a necessary exercise for mobility and flexibility. Because the legs are the largest extremities, they may take numerous stretches to reap the full benefits. The quadriceps muscle, which is located on the top part of your upper leg, is targeted in this exercise.

Standing Quadriceps Stretch

Before stretching, make sure you limber yourself by slowly walking around. As you will be balancing on one leg for this exercise, grab a chair or the back of a couch for support. The greater the weight of the support, the better.

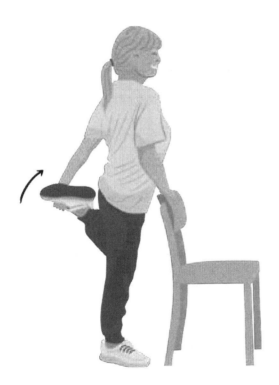

1. With your left hand, hold on to the chair.

2. Bend your right knee and grip your leg by the ankle with your right hand, gently pulling your foot toward your bottom.

3. Hold for 10 to 30 seconds before lowering and repeating with your left leg.

If you have trouble standing up, try this next one, which is also an excellent quadriceps stretch.

Seated Ankle Stretch

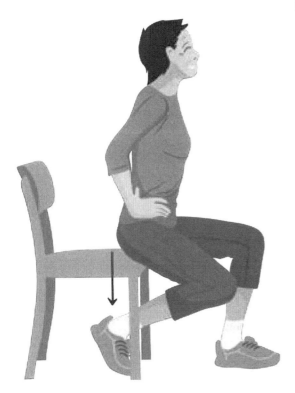

DIRECTIONS

1. Sit on the chair's front edge. There should be open space underneath the chair

2. Your right foot should be tucked under the chair.

3. Gently press down on your foot until you feel a stretch.

4. Hold the position for 20 to 30 seconds.

5. Then do the same thing with your left foot.

Seated Knee to Chest

This lower body stretch is essential for us seniors since it engages more than just our legs. The knee to chest stretching exercise increases hip and knee mobility by stretching the joints, as well as improving lower back flexibility. This stretch has the extra benefit of not requiring you to stand!

DIRECTIONS

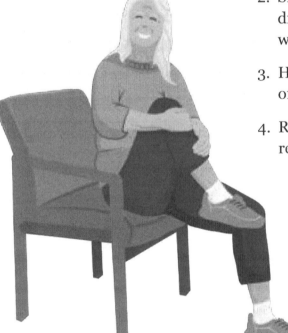

1. Warm-up your legs by walking, similar to the previous workout.

2. Sit comfortably in your chair and slowly draw your right knee toward your chest while seated.

3. Hold this position for 10 to 30 seconds once you feel the stretching sensation.

4. Return your leg to the floor gently and repeat the exercise with your other leg.

Hamstring Stretch

Now that we've taken care of your quadriceps and hips, it's time to focus on your hamstrings. This stretching exercise focuses on your lower back and legs, which are important for ensuring agility in seniors. It can help you stay mobile and fluid by reducing stiffness in your legs and back.

DIRECTIONS

1. Choose a solid surface to sit on.

2. Then, extend one of your legs on top of the surface.

3. Lean forward slowly, take a deep breath, and reach for your thigh, knee, or ankle. (Be careful not to hyperextend your hamstring when doing this stretch.)

4. Hold this position for 10 to 30 seconds before slowly lowering your leg and repeating with the opposite side of your body.

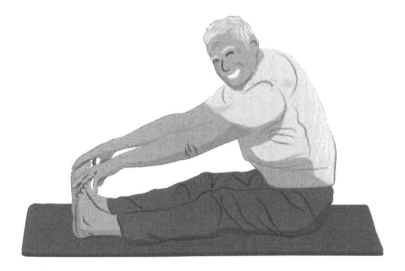

Soleus Stretch

Another major muscle group in your legs are the calve muscles, which can benefit greatly from this simple stretch. The soleus stretch improves the deep calve muscles and the overall functionality of your legs, which strengthens your calves and enhances lower body flexibility.

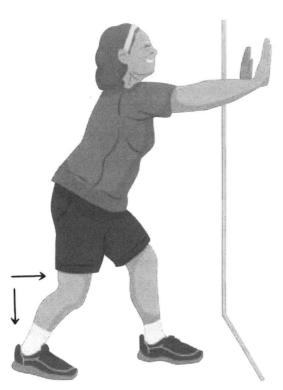

DIRECTIONS

1. Face a wall while standing upright.

2. Place your right foot in front of your left and support yourself by placing both hands on the wall in front of you.

3. Once you're comfortable, start bending your knees slowly until you feel a stretch in your lower thigh. For 10 to 30 seconds, stay in this position.

4. Slowly get up, switch the locations of your left and right feet, and repeat the exercise until you feel nice and stretched.

Upper Body Stretches:

We'll begin preparing the upper body now!

Overhead Side Stretches

The standing side stretch, also known as the overhead side stretch, is a simple and effective approach to loosening up your belly, back, and shoulders.

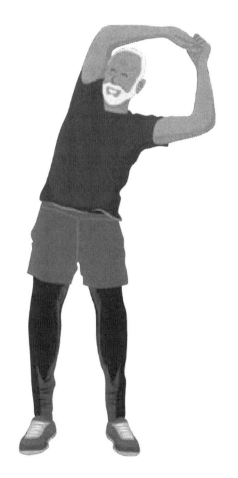

HO W TO:

1. Raise your arms over your head, interlocking your fingers if desired, with your feet shoulder-width apart.

2. Slowly lean to the left, keeping your torso long.

3. Return to the center after holding this position for 10 to 30 seconds; repeat the stretch on the right side.

Another benefit of this workout is that it may be done while sitting. So, for people who have issues with mobility, you can complete this exercise in the following steps:

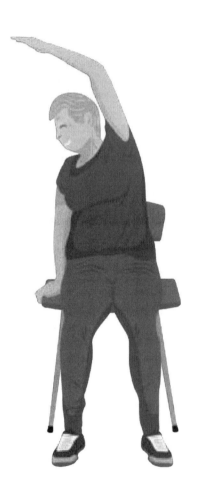

STEPS

1. Keep your hips, knees, and toes looking forward while sitting in an elevated chair.

2. Repeat the directions above with your arms raised over your head. (If this is too tough for you, put your arms on your hips or down by your sides.)

3. Lean gently to one side for 10 to 30 seconds.

Shoulder Stretch

We'll stick with the upper body for our next stretch and concentrate on the shoulders. You can open your shoulder joint with this basic shoulder stretch, which can help relieve muscle soreness and avoid deterioration.

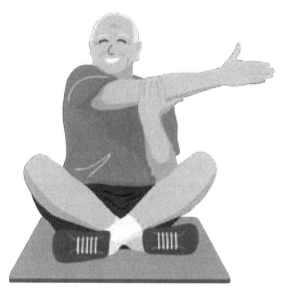

DIRECTIONS

1. Stand or sit as tall as you possibly can.

2. With your opposite hand, grab one of your arms and gently draw it across your chest until you feel a stretch in your shoulder. (While stretching, make sure your elbow stays below shoulder height.)

3. Hold this position for 10 to 30 seconds, then switch arms and repeat.

This stretch, like the one before it, can be done standing or sitting, depending on your preference for getting the most out of your stretching exercises.

Triceps Stretch

The triceps stretch is next on our list, and it's the final for our upper body. This stretch is a terrific method to enhance the mobility of your shoulders while stretching your arms. It can be done while standing or sitting, just like the rest of our upper body exercises. Remember to keep your back straight by sitting tall and using a chair!

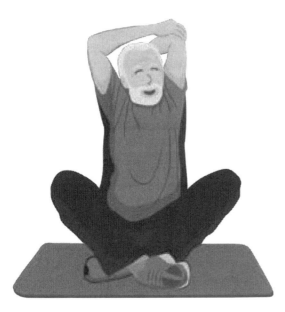

DIRECTIONS

1. Place your feet hip-width apart and stand (or sit) tall.

2. Raise both arms above your head, bending the right arm behind your head.

3. Then, using your left hand on your right elbow, slowly draw your elbow down toward your back until you feel your upper arm stretching.

4. Retain for 10 to 30 seconds, then return your arms to their original positions and repeat the stretch with your left arm.

Advanced Stretching Exercises

So far, we've covered a few muscle groups and learned a bit about your upper and lower bodies, but what about the middle? Because these more advanced stretches can be challenging, they are not required. Always listen to your body and only do this workout if you feel ready.

Lunge in a Chair

This hip stretch is ideal for seniors who want to preserve their mobility and muscle strength.

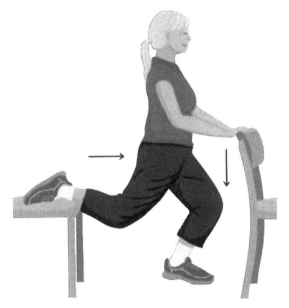

DIRECTIONS

1. Place two strong chairs approximately three feet apart facing the same direction.

2. Stand a few steps in front of the chair behind you and rest your shin on the chair's seat. With your foot dangling over the back of the chair, your knee should extend just past the front border.

3. Then, while moving your hips forward and down, slightly bend your front knee. Hold this position for 10 to 30 seconds before switching to the other side.

Standing Hip Flexor

The standing hip flexor stretch is last but not least on our list of senior stretches. This stretch, one of many hip flexor stretches for seniors, is a terrific technique to relieve hip tightness or pain. It should be emphasized, however, that this is a difficult exercise that is best suited for those with more experience.

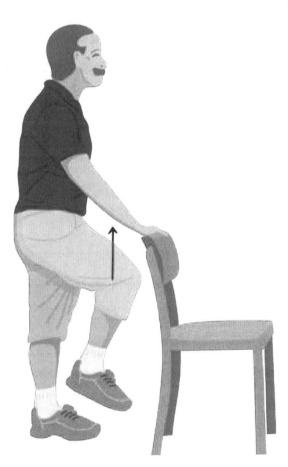

DIRECTIONS

1. To begin, take a strong chair and stand with your foot facing the chair's back, ensuring that you are far enough away from the chair to pull your leg up.

2. While holding both hands on the chair, keep one leg straight and elevate your opposite leg toward your chest with your knee bent as close to your chest as possible.

3. Stay in this position for 10 to 15 seconds before switching to the other leg.

We are almost at the end of this chapter, and I want to end it on an important note. Have you ever noticed that once you create a routine of stretching on a regular basis, you ultimately fall out of the habit and stop stretching altogether? Since stretching does not result in a visible change in our appearance, we tend to overlook the necessity of these simple exercises. However, if not done correctly, most likely these stretches will not benefit you at all. In fact, when done wrong and on the wrong patient (for example someone doing an advanced stretch they are not ready for) they can cause muscle injury.[4]

We must begin to consider mobility in a much broader context. We need to start thinking about our long-term health. Flexibility does not manifest itself in the form of more muscular arms or a toned tummy, and you won't leave feeling like you've had a good workout. However, proper flexibility gained via regular stretching can allow you to use your body in new ways and keep you moving effectively for the rest of your life. It's also important to remember that better mobility is one of the vital achievements of any exercise routine. Our quest for a better, fitter, healthier, and injury/pain-free self begins with more ease of movement. So, start by putting "increasing flexibility" at the top of your priority list and stretching regularly to keep your movements at an optimal level.

References:

1. Smith, CA. (1994). The warm-up procedure: To stretch or not to stretch. A brief review. *Journal of Orthopaedic and Sports Physical Therapy*, 19: 12–17

2. Cross, KM., & Worrell, TW. (1999). Effects of a static stretching program on the incidence of lower extremity musculotendinous strains. *Journal of Athletic Training*, 34(1): 11–14.

3. Micheo, W., Baerga, L., & Miranda, G. (2012). Basic principles regarding strength, flexibility, and stability exercises. *PM & R: The journal of injury, function, and rehabilitation*, 4(11), 805–811.

4. Shrier, I. (2005). When and whom to stretch? Gauging the benefits and drawbacks for individual patients. *The Physician and Sports Medicine,* 33(3): 22–26.

Chapter 4: Core Strength is Critical

"Some people are old at 18 and some are young at 90..
time is a concept that humans created "

Yoko Ono

Core muscles: If you knew nothing about them before starting your exercise, then it's no wonder why you can't get your balance and strength back with your previous exercise routines. Core muscles are the most basic muscles, which act as the anchors of your body to keep it grounded. As you know by now, muscles have a lot of functions apart from giving strength. The intricate push and pull of several muscle groups is what moves our limbs, controls our posture, and gives us balance. Weak muscles may not always mean that you have a weak grip or can't lift heavy things. More often than not, weak muscles translate into bad posture, poor gait, and loss of balance.

It is a mistake that people make all the time, thinking if they can lift a chair or carry their own bags, they have decent strength in their muscles. Obviously, that's not correct. There are several reasons why. The first reason is that muscles are not interconnected. Muscle health depends on how much nutrition and exercise those muscles receive. The muscles you regularly use, for example your forearm muscle (if you write every day), will get more blood supply and become thicker. In the meantime, another one of your muscles, on your torso or legs, can become very weak and shrink in size. When you do workouts that do nothing for your core muscles, the same thing happens. You may end up having well-developed biceps, while having weak abdominal and back muscles.

What are the Core Muscles?

Your core is composed of your abdominals, hips, back, and chest. These are called "core" because they are situated around the central area of your body and control much of the balance and weight distribution. Although the concept of core muscles is an anatomic or medical one, most exercises don't follow the textbook definition of it. Interestingly enough, you can find a lot of different theories and ideas of which muscles should be considered as "core." According to sports physicians," The core is the musculature that surrounds the lumbopelvic region and includes the abdominals anteriorly, the paraspinals and glutes posteriorly, the pelvic floor musculature inferiorly, the hip abductors and rotators laterally, and diaphragm superiorly" (Bliss & Teeple, 2005)[1]. Think of the core as a box that surrounds your torso, with the abdomen on the front, the spine and the buttocks on the back, the pelvic floor below and the diaphragm on top. So, the core muscles surround the center of gravity and center of rotation of your body.

The core muscles work to stabilize your body, allowing for a greater range of movement and improving balance. The importance of core muscles is well established among physiotherapists. We get to that later, but let's learn what the core muscles are first:

- **Rectus Abdominis (six-pack muscle):** This pair of muscles is attached to the central part of the 5th to 7th ribs and the tip of the sternum. Its pri- mary movement is bringing the diaphragm toward the pelvis, like when you sit up in bed or do a crunch. It flexes the spine at the lower back region.

- **Internal and External Obliques:** These attach on the lateral side of your trunk, connecting the pubis and the iliac bone to the ribs. Their primary movements involve trunk rotation (like turning to look over your shoulder) and side bending.

- **Transverse Abdominis:** This pair of muscles attaches from the lower spine under the ribs and around the body to the rectus abdominis. As the deepest of the abdominal muscles, they tighten and support the spine and abdomen. This important pair of muscles often controls the shape of the abdomen. Especially in women after pregnancy, the transverse muscles can become very weak.

- **Pelvic floor:** These muscles attach to the underside of the pelvis. Having a weak pelvic floor prevents you from doing heavy lifting or heavy work where you need to take strength from the abdomen. The pelvic floor works as a barrier in keeping the abdominal pressure in control and the contents from pushing into the pelvic cavity.

- **Diaphragm:** The diaphragm separates the chest cavity from the abdominal cavity. It also keeps the abdominal pressure within itself. The diaphragm is responsible for breathing in and out. As it contracts, it flattens, allowing room for the lungs to expand. When it relaxes, it compresses the lung cavity and forces air out.

- **Erector spinae:** These muscles keep the back straight and help rotate it.

Why are Core Muscle Exercises Important?

Core muscles control the way you hold and move your body. Naturally, with aging, our core muscles (along with other muscles) get weaker. On top of that, most people get very little to zero core muscle exercise in their adult lives. We all like to think that the little exercise we do now and then has a lasting effect. However, the body is always changing. Doing exercise sparingly, even heavy exercise, does not benefit your core. That is why most of us have weak cores and backaches, despite working out now and then.

When done regularly and correctly, core exercises target the muscles in your lower body (pelvis and hips), lower back, and abdomen, building muscular connections that encourage the muscles to work better together. When these muscles are working together and are exercised regularly, you'll also be less susceptible to injuries, and it will lower the strain on your muscles and joints. That's because your body will be staying in alignment more naturally. It will also heal the existing damages to the tissues and nerves in that area. Which leads to a good portion of your chronic pain going away.

The efficacy of core exercise is surprising. If you are someone who has been suffering from chronic pain, you know that it is hard to treat with just medications or even surgery—even those have lasting side effects. There is no permanent treatment. So, naturally, doctors recommend safer treatment options like exercise, yoga, meditation, etc. Several pieces of research have been conducted to find which pains and to what extent these exercises can help with, and they all reported amazing results!

I am sure you know at least a dozen people who have tried to exercise and get healthier but failed to do so. I mean, how many people join gyms and yoga classes and return with zero benefits? Does that mean the exercises don't work? No, they do. People who fail to achieve their goal, whether that be mobility or pain relief, with exercise are simply following the wrong prescriptions! In fact, there was a study which showed that the elderly who were prescribed more exercise done more often don't necessarily have their expectations met. This is due to a lack of clear guidelines. How are you supposed to know which exercise to do? As we have discussed earlier, there is no simple one-size-fits-all routine when it comes to exercising. You need to know what your target muscles are in order to fix them. Often, we go in blind, and for that reason, we see no results at all. Thus, knowing about and practicing core exercises are important.

The core supports your entire body. The back and abdomen basically support your spine and the weight of your torso. If you have weak back muscles, it pushes weight into the lower back muscles and hip joints. This leads to muscle strains, vertebral disc degeneration, hip fractures, and back pain. Back pain is common these days due to long sitting hours and less exercise. In fact, four out of five Americans suffer from lower back pain.

The good news is that researchers have found improving core strength can help eliminate back pain. This research was done on thirty patients undergoing treatment by the National Institute for the Orthopaedically Handicapped in India. After treating half of the subjects with core muscle exercises, the doctors reassessed their situation. The results of the study showed that, in only six weeks, there was a significant improvement in the patients' conditions. The researchers concluded that, "Core muscle strengthening exercise along with lumbar flexibility and gluteus maximus strengthening is an effective rehabilitation technique for all chronic low back pain patients irrespective of duration (less than one year and more than one year) of their pain" (Kumar et al., 2015)[2]. And this is not the only study. Other research on core muscle exercises also shows them to be a highly successful method of treatment.

Strong core muscles mean you can go about your day with ease. You can walk comfortably and do most physical activities without having to depend on anyone, including reaching for things on high shelves, cleaning the car, and bending down to tie your shoes. Here are some everyday tasks that require a healthy core:

In the Office

It makes sense that jobs involving lifting, twisting and standing all rely on core muscles, but even sitting at your desk engages your core. In fact, sitting is probably the only time when we use our core muscles constantly over an extended period. When you are working on the computer, even though you are using only your hands, the muscles of the back of your neck and back of the chest provides support. Without proper core exercises, you will feel the strain in your back and shoulders.

At Home

Everyday tasks like turning to look behind you, sitting in a chair, or just standing still all involve engaging your core. Cooking requires both upper body muscles and core muscles. If you want to cook for your family, you need to lift heavy pots and pans. Of course, you will also need to cut with a knife, stir with spoons, etc. (These all require fine motor skills that we will talk about later). Good posture lessens wear and tear on the spine and allows you to do simple housework like mopping the floor, dusting, cleaning the shelves, fixing the furniture, etc. For people who live alone, this is especially beneficial. You must depend on yourself during emergencies like storms, blackouts, or even broken pipes. Having a strong core means you can easily reach down and fix that leaking pipe or pick your own tomatoes from the garden.

Engaging in Hobbies

Retirement is the perfect time for hobbies. Most people, after retirement, start their own hobbies they couldn't find time for before. For example, I enjoy gardening. Having a strong core will leave you free to choose from a wide array of hobbies like gardening, sculpting, rowing, and even biking. Once you realize there is no limit to what you can or cannot do, you will enjoy trying new things every week.

How do I Build a Strong Core?

Because many people associate the core with only abdominal muscles, they think that core strengthening just means doing ab workouts and targeting those muscles. However, as you've learned, you also need to be training your hips and back while learning how to stabilize all of your core muscles. A few of the classic core exercises can hurt instead of help. Two exercises, in particular, have a high risk of injury—crunches and traditional sit-ups. These moves put a lot of pressure on the spine, making it easy to injure yourself.

Exercises

After all that talk, you must be wondering about the exercises. Well, here are a few core exercises you can do at home:

- planks
- sit-ups
- bridges
- bird dogs

Except for these, there are other simple exercises you can do as well. One of the quick ones is an abdominal draw. While other exercises will be covered in later chapters, let's take a look at this simple exercise, so you can try it right now.

Abdominal Draw

DIRECTIONS

1. Lie on your back with your knees bent or sit up straight in a chair.

2. Suck in your stomach, imagining that you are drawing your belly button to your spine.

3. You should be able to breathe normally but will feel the muscles around your abdomen and sides tighten. Make sure your back is straight and isn't pushing into the ground.

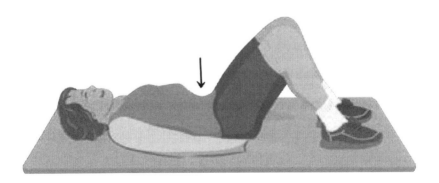

4. Hold for 5-10 seconds, relax, then repeat.

Try doing his exercise a few times. You can also skip to chapter 6 to get more core exercises if you want to start right away.

References:

1. Bliss, L. S., & Teeple, P. (2005). Core stability: the centerpiece of any training program. Current sports medicine reports, 4(3), 179-183.

2. Kumar, T., Kumar, S., Nezamuddin, M., & Sharma, V. P. (2015). Efficacy of core muscle strengthening exercise in chronic low back pain patients. Journal of back and musculoskeletal rehabilitation, 28(4), 699-707.

Chapter 5: Strength Training is not Just for Gym Rats!

If you go into almost any gym in the US, you will find people lifting weights in the corner like it's nobody's business. There will always be people who love getting "jacked." They do all kinds of strength training, take protein shakes, dehydrate themselves, and whatnot. While it's not a bad thing, getting 6 pack is not the goal of most people over 60. So, most of us stay away from the dumbbells and the pull-up bars and stick to the treadmill. What if I told you that these muscle-making exercises have some use to us after all?

You may not know this, but strength training, when done correctly, is beneficial for everyone. A workout routine without strength training is like a table missing a leg—incomplete and prone to collapse. Strength training keeps your muscles strong, reverses muscle loss due to age, and improves bone health and joint mobility. It's not just about gaining strength; it's about improving your balance, your stamina, and overall health.

Strength training is also known as resistance training. This means, the individual works against resistance or force while moving their bodies. This is comparatively different from regular training. In regular workouts like jumping jacks or running, you work with only your body weight. The energy you are spending, and the "work" your muscles are doing are against your own weight. For example, if you weigh about 150 pounds, when you are doing yoga or running, you are working with a fraction of 150 pounds. It doesn't feel too difficult because the muscles that make up much of the weight are themselves moving, and you are only working with part of your weight. So, if you are of moderate weight, the forces "resisting" or acting against your movements are also moderate, and there is no way to control or increase the resistance force.

On the other hand, in resistance training, you are working with weights, springs, or non-moving objects. As you do the workouts, there will be extra "resistance" or forces acting against your movements. Hence, when you are doing resistance workouts, your muscles must overcome those forces. As a result, they need to work more. As I probably have mentioned before, muscle cells can and do increase in size and number as you work them more. These neat little traits that nature has bestowed upon us are called hypertrophy and hyperplasia. These two mechanisms (along with atrophy which is their opposite) help humans and animals adapt to their unique environments. For example, someone who works at a construction site has muscular arms because they lift a lot, and their muscles need to be strong to handle the extra work. People who work with mainly their right/left hands, pitchers or archers, usually have more muscles in that respective hand as well. The point of resistance training is that by using this theory, you can reverse the loss of muscle strength.

Resistance training can be immensely helpful for people of advanced age. With aging, we tend to lose muscle mass and control. It's a phenomenon called sarcopenia (Deschenes et al., 2021)[1]. This significant increase in disability, frailty, and falls with advancing age is a problem. Strength training has long been proven to be effective against this problem, regardless of age or gender. There is a good amount of research to prove it as well. One study, for example, was done on 12 individuals between the ages of 60 and 72 years. They all did strength exercises, like knee extensions and leg curls, and followed a standard prescription of three sets of eight repetitions for three days per week. After 12 WEeks, their strength was at 150%, with a 10% increase in muscle mass (Frontera et al., n.d.)[2]. Other similar studies show an increase in strength by 150%, in gait speed by 48%, balance by 14%, and a reduction of physical and overall disability by 15 - 18% (Seguin & Nelson, 2003)[3].

Although many of these benefits are well known, we most often only see people who are already somewhat fit doing these exercises. This is because of the common misconception that strength training is only for those who are in good health. While it's true that you need to have at least some strength and balance before starting resistance exercises, there is no reason more people cannot do them. In fact, someone who is suffering from chronic pain or mobility issues benefits substantially from resistance exercises. This is especially true for chronic conditions like stroke, multiple sclerosis, osteoarthritis, chronic back pain, chronic heart failure Research has shown that after only 8 weeks of strength exercises, patients with systemic sclerosis managed to improve their lower extremity strength, ambulatory function, fatigue, and overall quality of life (White et al., 2004)[4]. Other studies showed similar results for patients with heart diseases and neurodegenerative diseases. A very recent study, done in 2021, even showed that among adults with intellectual disability, strength exercise can be used successfully for empowerment—by promoting muscular strength and independent functional performance (Obrusnikova et al., 2001)[5]. These benefits are extraordinary considering how strength exercises are usually associated with getting slim or gaining heavy muscles. As I have shown you, that is clearly not the case.

Types of Strength Training

If you are new to strength training, it can be a little intimidating, especially for those of us with little or no fitness background. Even if you had an interest in strength training before, a quick google image search can scare you away. Having scared myself by that very thing, I would advise against it! Jokes aside, strength training is so much more than dropping barbells or straining with heavy weights. Based on the type of resistance, there are two types of strength training:

- **Isometric Resistance:** In this type of strength training, you are contracting your muscles against a non-moving object, like pushing against the floor in a pushup. Here, the force you apply through your hands transfers back to your body; thus, you are moving your body off the floor or up the pull-up bar.

- **Isotonic Strength Training:** In these exercises, you are contracting your muscles through a range of motions, like in weightlifting. So, you are moving your body and an object as well.

With the risk of sounding like a broken record, let me mention again that muscles work by the "use it or lose it" principle. Those that go neglected will become weak, and your lean muscle mass will naturally diminish as you get older. This means your body fat percentage will increase over time if you don't put in the effort to replace the lost lean muscle. As the weight of fat is less than muscle, it is difficult to catch muscle loss with the naked eye. You may look the same but still lose muscle mass. It also means that you can lose weight but gain fat at the same time. This often happens as people try to lose weight without workouts. They aim to lose weight but lose muscle mass instead.

Strength training will help you preserve and enhance muscle mass while losing fat. As this type of training burns a lot of calories, you will be using a good portion of your fat reserve while doing this. This is good news for the arteries, of course, but also for you! You will finally be able to move the way you want. However, we will not jump directly into training with weights. Instead, you'll want to start by focusing on form and establishing a base level of strength. There's no need to start with confusing-looking equipment and heavyweights just yet. We will take a safer approach.

We will start with functional movements that include lifting, pushing, pulling, etc. These movements are done with bodyweight (or other weights as you progress) to give you the extra load that will build muscle and coordination.

All strength exercises should be approached this way. Start small and work your way up. Don't try to do the difficult ones first, and obviously, don't take on too heavy of a weight at first. Here are a few things to use as part of strength training:

- bodyweight
- resistance tubing/resistance bands
- free weights
- weight machines
- cable suspension training
- If you do not have access to these, you can use other things lying in the house like water bottles, canned food, etc.

Here are some exercises you can do as part of your strength training:

- seated shoulder press
- push-up
- leg curl
- lunge
- single-arm dumbbell row
- squat

Benefits of Strength Training

- **Develop strong bones:** According to a recent study published in the Journal of Aging and Health, a resistance exercise session three times per week improved bone density, structure, and strength in postmenopausal women without hormone replacement therapy (Bocalini et al., 2009)[6].

- **Manage your weight:** All exercise helps boost your metabolism, meaning your body burns calories more efficiently. Strength training helps weight loss more than aerobic exercise because it keeps your metabolism active for longer. The more muscle mass you have, the more calories you'll burn.

- **Enhance Quality of Life:** Strength training improves balance, coordination, and posture. This also helps reduce the chances of falling.

- **Manage Chronic Conditions:** Conditions like arthritis, back pain, obesity, heart disease, depression, and diabetes are all improved with the right exercise.

- **Increase Mental Acuity:** Some research shows that strength training and aerobic exercise may improve thinking and learning skills for older adults.

- **Boost energy levels and mood:** Exercise increases endorphins—chemicals that trigger positive feelings.

Strength training is important. However, it is equally important to rest. At any age, the first rule to exercise is be safe. So, take a day or two off in between sessions. Three days per week is perfectly adequate! If you want to do strength training a few days in a row, target different muscle groups each day, so that each group has time to recover between sessions.

References:

1. Deschenes, M. R., Oh, J., & Tufts, H. (2021). The role of the neuromuscular junction in sarcopenia. In sarcopenia (pp. 59-80). Elsevier.

2. Frontera W, Merideth C, O'Reilly K, Knuttgen H, Evans W. (n.d.). Strength conditioning in older men: skeletal muscle hypertrophy and improved function. J Appl Physiol 1988;64.

3. Seguin, R., & Nelson, M. E. (2003). The benefits of strength training for older adults. American journal of preventive medicine, 25(3), 141-149.

4. White, L. J., McCoy, S. C., Castellano, V., Gutierrez, G., Stevens, J. E., Walter, G. A., & Vandenborne, K. (2004). Resistance training improves strength and

functional capacity in persons with multiple sclerosis. Multiple sclerosis journal, 10(6), 668-674.

5. Obrusnikova, I., Cavalier, A. R., Suminski, R. R., Blair, A. E., Firkin, C. J., & Steinbrecher, A. M. (2021). A resistance training intervention for adults with intellectual disability in the community: A pilot randomized clinical trial. Adapted Physical Activity Quarterly, 1(Aop), 1-23.

6. Bocalini, D. S., Serra, A. J., dos Santos, L., Murad, N., & Levy, R. F. (2009). Strength training preserves the bone mineral density of postmenopausal women without hormone replacement therapy. Journal of Aging and Health, 21(3), 519-527.

Chapter 5: Strength Training is not Just for Gym Rats

Chapter 6: 21 Bodyweight Exercises in 21 days

Having good health and a great body shape sounds wonderful, but it is quite difficult to achieve. Most assume it's because of the physical difficulty of the exercises or the busy life we lead. Some would even say it's because of the food we eat. However, the real reason is pretty simple. It is hard to stick to an exercise routine!

Make it a Habit

It's not just you! Most people have difficulty following their exercise routines. Creating any habit is difficult, not just exercise. A habit is successfully formed when you are so used to doing something, you do it unconsciously. To reach that level, you have to pass a few stages. There is a lot of science behind this, but I won't bore you with that, so let's jump straight into the steps.

Step 1

The first step is to start. It's easy to avoid beginning a new routine even after you have everything planned out. You cannot build a daily habit until you begin. Plan a day when you will start, and don't deviate. Promise yourself you will start exercising no matter what.

Step 2

The next step is to make exercising a non-negotiable part of your life. To do that, set a time for exercising every day. Yes, you read that right. You need to do something daily to really make it a part of your life. Repeat it enough times and it comes to you unconsciously. This part is the hardest. You will not always want to, nor will you always have time for exercising. This is expected. After all, you are trying to fit something new into your daily life. It will be an inconvenience at first, but you must be resilient. Below are a few techniques to help make this step easier:

- Schedule your exercise early in the morning before brushing your teeth. That way, you won't be able to put it off later.

- Find a group of friends or create a community group to do the workouts with you. Having someone else hold you accountable is a good way to stay on track.

- Set a daily alarm during your exercise time.

- Get a fitness app. There are plenty of free apps in the apple or android stores that will help you stay motivated. These often have reminders, timers, motivational quotes, and scoring systems as well. You will have fun using these.

Step 3

The next step is to make the process more enjoyable. No matter how much scheduling you do, you won't do something you hate every day. It will just make you miserable. The key to building a habit is to make it enjoyable. Even if you don't enjoy the whole thing, try to bring in some elements that you do like. For example, you can buy comfortable or cute workout gear or make a pretty exercise corner in your home with plush rugs and soothing music. The point is, working out should not make you stressed or unhappy; instead, it should be relaxing. Find what you like and do that!

Even with the best intentions, you may face some difficulties. The best way to overcome those is to have a solid routine to follow. Without that, you will most likely do the same exercises every day and miss out on a more rounded workout.

The Routine

To help get things rolling, start with some basic exercises and move on to the hard ones from there. Over the next 21 days (three weeks), you're going to perform a different bodyweight exercise each day. By the time that we are done, you'll find that you're more comfortable with your form, and the moves will start to feel familiar to you.

For each of these moves, aim for 1-3 sets of 8-12 repetitions each. Increase as you become more comfortable with the moves and your strength increases. You only need 15 minutes.

The format for these workouts will be as follows:

1. 5 minutes of warm-up exercises like walking

2. 5 minutes of stretching

3. 5 minutes of the exercise for the day

If you find that you finish before the five minutes are up, go back to the exercise from the previous day.

Week 1

Day 1: Wall Pushups

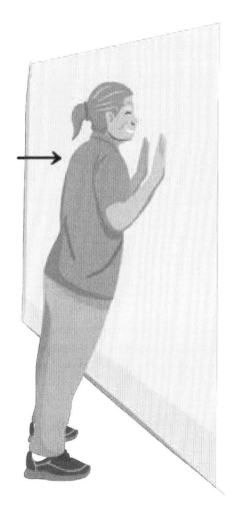

DIRECTIONS

1. Stand up and face a wall or any vertical surface; keep 1.5 to 2 feet in distance.

2. Put your hands to the wall, keeping them straight; the distance between your elbow and shoulders should be the same.

3. Bend your elbows diagonally and bring your chest closer to the wall.

4. Using your forearms, press into the wall again in a pushing motion and get back to the original standing position. You can let your heels lift off the floor if that's more comfortable.

   Modification: the closer you are to the wall, the easier this move will be.

Day 2: Chair Squats/Sit to Stands

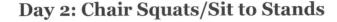

DIRECTIONS

1. Stand straight with a chair behind you (like you usually would before sitting).

2. Bend your knees to lower yourself onto the chair, touching the chair only briefly with your bottom.

3. Stand back up using your thighs and legs.

Modification: Using the same technique, sit all the way down in the chair. Then, use your legs and arms to power your movement back up to standing.

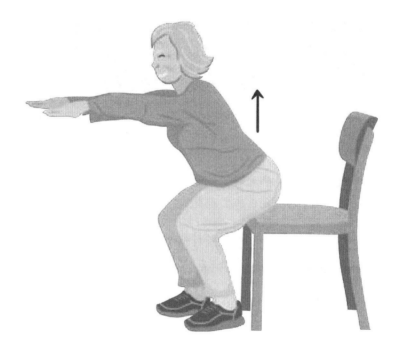

Day 3: Glute Bridge

DIRECTIONS

1. Lie on your back with your knees bent and your feet flat on the floor about hip-width apart.

2. Press your arms to the floor, and push through your feet, squeezing your glutes to raise your hips into the air.

3. Once your body forms a straight line, pause, then slowly lower back down to your starting position.

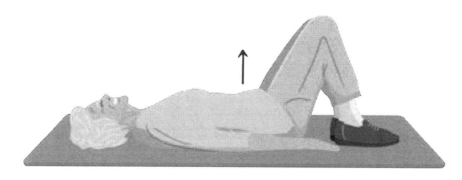

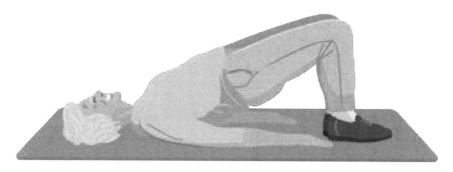

Day 4: Squats

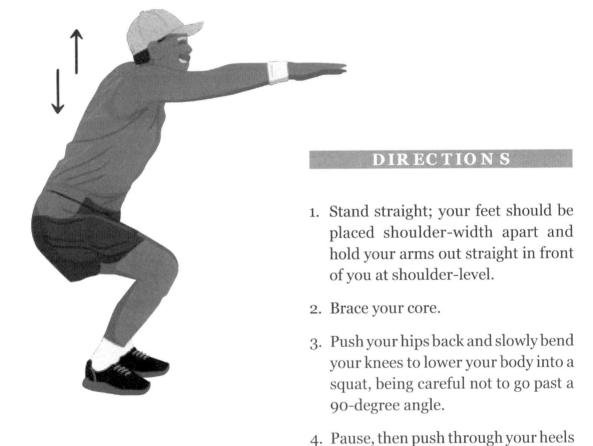

DIRECTIONS

1. Stand straight; your feet should be placed shoulder-width apart and hold your arms out straight in front of you at shoulder-level.

2. Brace your core.

3. Push your hips back and slowly bend your knees to lower your body into a squat, being careful not to go past a 90-degree angle.

4. Pause, then push through your heels to return to the starting position

Day 5: Wall Angels

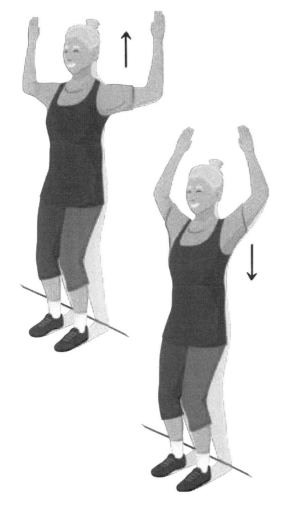

DIRECTIONS

1. Stand with your back on the wall without leaning on it. Your feet should be a few inches away from the wall; otherwise, you'll fall.

2. While keeping your head touching the wall and your arms down by your sides, look straight forward so the back of your head is touching the wall (you may feel some discomfort in your neck doing this, but no worries, it's normal).

3. Bend your legs a little to really push your body against the wall.

4. Then, put your arms beside your head, palms up, and elbow flush to the wall in a surrender position.

5. Raise your arms as high as you can while maintaining proper form and lower your arms back to start.

   *Stop if you feel discomfort.

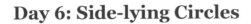

Day 6: Side-lying Circles

1. Lie on your side. Use a floor mat or carpet to avoid hurting your pelvic bones.

2. Position your body in a straight line with your bottom arm extended straight past your head.

3. Bend the elbow of the other hand and place the palm on the floor in front of your chest.

4. Resting your head on your bottom arm, squeeze your abdominals to pull in your stomach.

5. Lift your left leg to about hip height and move your leg in small clockwise circles. Pause, then repeat in a counterclockwise motion. Don't move it too fast or high, or you can make the lower back pain worse.

6. Lower your leg, then repeat the other side.

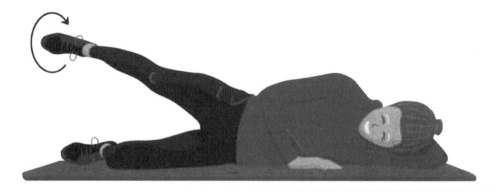

Note: be sure to keep your hips directly over one another when performing this move

Day 7: Standing Marches

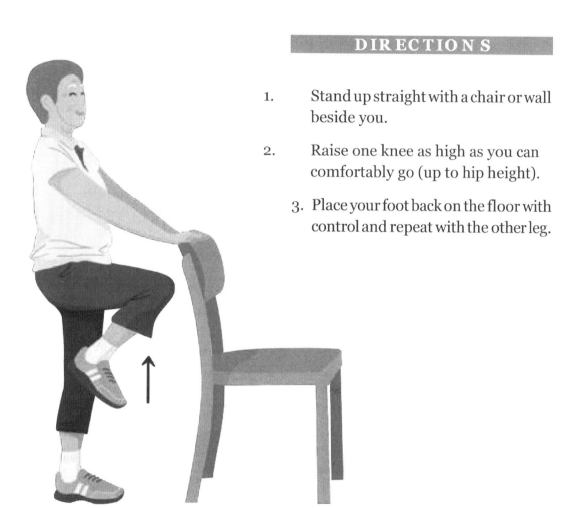

DIRECTIONS

1. Stand up straight with a chair or wall beside you.

2. Raise one knee as high as you can comfortably go (up to hip height).

3. Place your foot back on the floor with control and repeat with the other leg.

Week 2

Day 8: Wall Slides

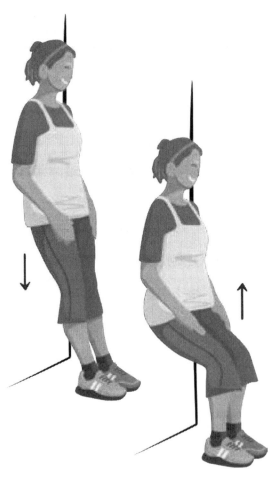

1. Stand with your back 1-2 feet away from the wall with your feet straight forward and sturdily placed on the ground.

2. Lean back on the wall so that your back, shoulders, butt, arms, and head are all flush with the wall; hold onto a chair for balance if needed.

3. Slowly bend your knees and slide down on the wall as much as you can while keeping the weight on your thighs and legs.

4. Hold this position for three counts before raising back up.

Do not go too low, or you can seriously hurt your knees.

Day 9: Standing Balance

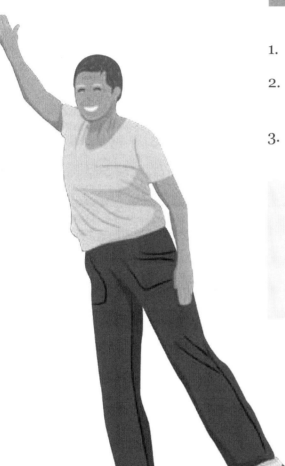

DIRECTIONS

1. Hold onto a steady surface.

2. Lift up one foot, balancing on the other for as long as you can.

3. Repeat on the other side.

Note: You'll eventually work up to standing on one foot without using the support and maintain that pose for a minute or longer

Day 10: Arm Circles

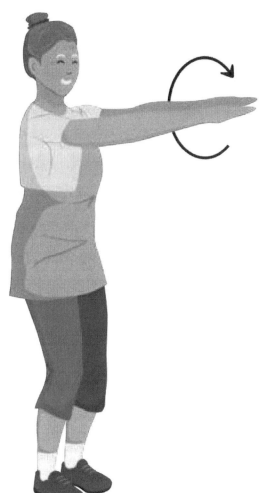

DIRECTIONS

1. Stand with your arms raised straight in front of your body.

2. With your arms ups, slowly move them in a clockwise circle of about 1 foot in diameter for 20-30 seconds.

3. Reverse the movement.

Day 11: Side Leg Lifts

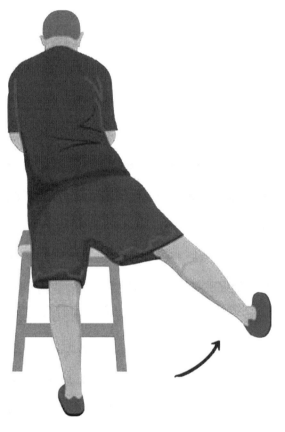

DIRECTIONS

1. Stand straight; your feet should be hip width apart, holding onto the back of a chair.

2. Shift your weight to one leg and raise the other leg laterally (to the side) as high as is comfortable.

3. Touch your toe back to the ground and lift the same leg again.

4. Repeat on both sides.

Modification: Carry out exercise as described but raise your leg behind you instead of laterally. Be sure to do this with control to avoid straining your lower back.

Day 12: Bird Dog

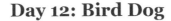

DIRECTIONS

1. Sit down on a comfortable mat and lean forward on your hands.

2. Put your weight on your knees and palms with your hands directly under your shoulders.

3. Tighten your stomach muscles and keep your back flat.

4. Keep your head straight and lift one hand to reach straight in front of your shoulder while lifting the opposite foot straight behind your hip. Your arm, leg, and body should all follow one straight line.

5. Hold this position for 6 seconds (or as long as you can stay balanced) then lower your hand and legs.

6. Then repeat on the opposite side.

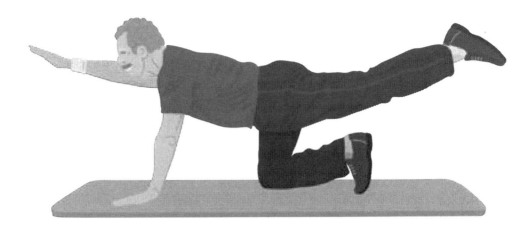

Day 13: Plank

DIRECTIONS

1. Lie down on a mat with your forearms on the floor and your hands clasped together.

2. Extend your legs straight out behind you, pushing up onto your toes.

3. Hold your back straight and tighten your core, holding the position for 30-60 seconds (or as long as is doable for you).

Modification: Extend your legs behind you, but instead of pushing onto your toes, lift your body from the knees up. This may be an easier way to accomplish this move until you build up more core strength.

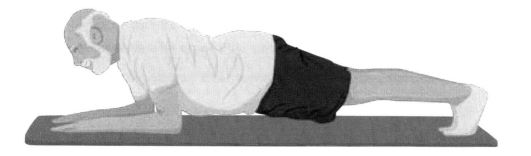

Day 14: Lunge

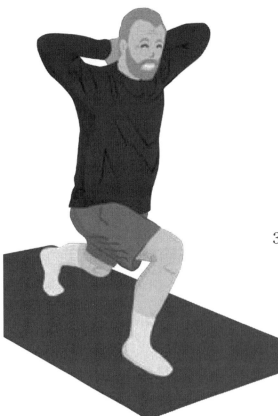

1. Stand near a wall or chair for balance with your feet hip-width apart, and hands on your hips.

2. Step your right leg forward and lower your body until your left knee is close to/touching the floor. The knee and thighs should be at 90 degrees with the body.

3. Stand up and repeat on the other side.

Modification: if you can't comfortably go down far enough to get your back knee at a 90-degree angle, go as far as is comfortable

Week 3

Day 15: Wall Sit

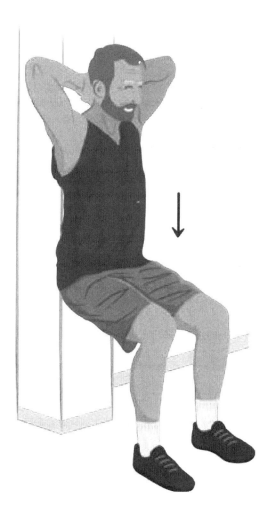

DIRECTIONS

1. Lean back against a wall and slowly slide your back down it until your thighs are parallel to the floor. Your knees should be directly above your ankles, and your back should be straight.

2. Hold for 30-60 seconds.

Day 16: Step-ups

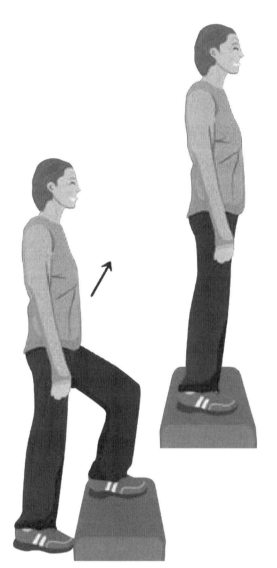

DIRECTIONS

1. Using stairs or a sturdy box, raise one foot onto the step.

2. Raise the other foot, so both feet are resting on the step.

3. Lower one foot back to the floor, then the other foot.

4. Complete one set using the same starting foot and switch.

Day 17: Single-leg Deadlift

DIRECTIONS

1. Get in a standing position and keep your feet together, with a chair or wall near you for support.

2. Put your body weight on one leg, keep it firm on the ground, and lean forward.

3. Move your leg back in the air (knees unbent) like a pendulum and, with your opposite hand, reach toward the ground. You can use both arms to reach toward the ground too. Try to get as close to the floor as you can.

4. Hold this position for 6 seconds and then slowly raise your torso while lowering your right leg and switching legs.

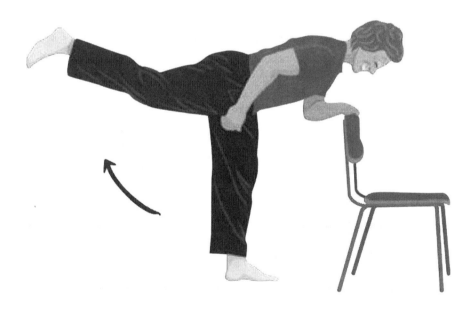

Day 18: Quadruped Leg Lift

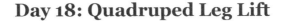

DIRECTIONS

1. Get on the ground and put your weight on your elbows, forearms, and knees, with your back flat and core engaged.

2. Raise your left leg straight back until your foot is at hip level and your thigh is parallel to the floor.

3. Balance as long as you can, then raise your bottom right toe off the floor. You should be tightening your butt, back, and abs with this move.

4. Hold for 10-20 seconds and switch legs.

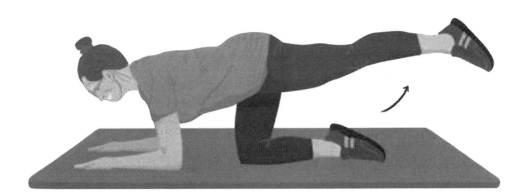

Day 19: Inchworm

1. Stand up tall with your legs straight.

2. Lean forward and slowly lower your torso toward the floor, placing your hands on the floor.

3. Move your hands forward (as if you are walking with them) until you are in a pushup position.

4. Start taking small steps forward with your feet until your feet meet your hands.

Note: make sure you don't lock your knees when performing this move. If you feel dizzy, you can skip the walking part and just hold the inversed "u" position for 6 seconds.

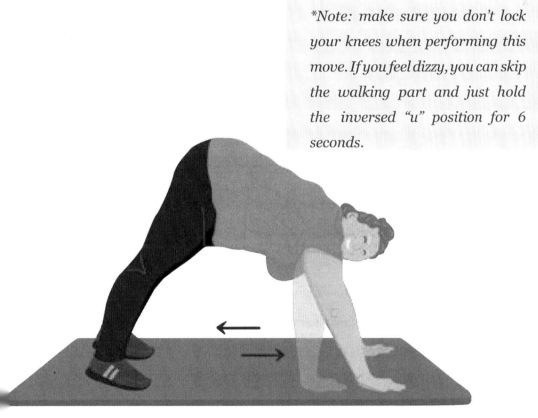

Day 20: Seated Twists

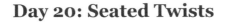

DIRECTIONS

1. Sit in a chair with your back straight and extended.

2. Raise your hands to a 90-degree angle from your body.

3. Keeping your lower body stationary, slowly rotate your torso to each side

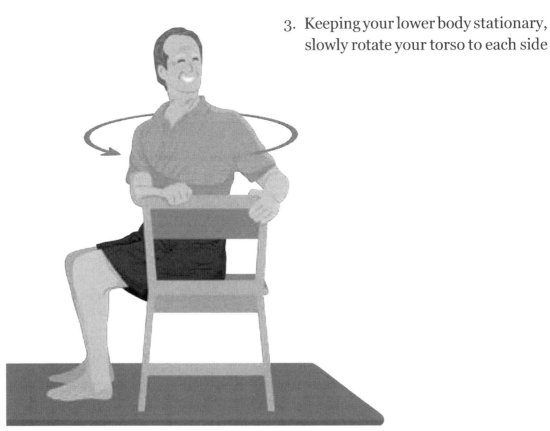

Day 21: Side Planks

DIRECTIONS

1. Lie on your right side with your right elbow taking your weight and your palms on your ears, propping you up.

2. With the sides of your feet stacked against one another, squeeze your core and lift your hips off the ground. Your body should be placed in a straight line from your ears to your feet.

3. Hold for 30-60 seconds or as long as possible.

4. Lower your hips and repeat on the left side

Modification: If you can't hold a plank with your feet stacked, you can stack (press together) the sides of your knees. This reduces the amount of weight you need to hold up.

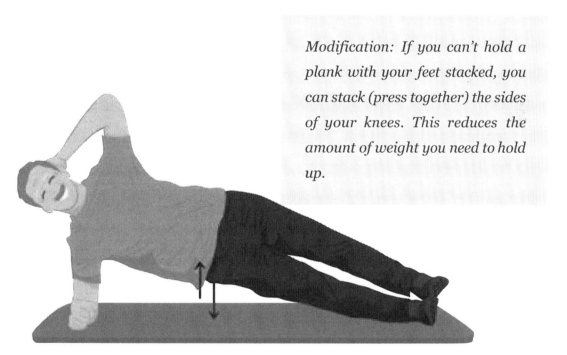

96

After following this routine for 21 days, you will feel more comfortable doing exercises. This routine is intended to get your body in the habit of exercising and performing basic day-to-day movements. After you have mastered the workouts mentioned here, you can create your own routine with the workouts you like best. However, I would suggest keeping some core exercises and weighted exercises 2-3 days per week in your new routine.

Chapter 7: 21 Strength Training Moves

After you have mastered the basic exercise routine, you can move on to the weighted exercise! For these, we will not follow the same method and do weighted exercises for 21 days at a stretch; rather, we will incorporate weighted exercises in between regular exercises to make a complete and well-rounded workout plan.

For the following exercises, aim to complete 1-2 sets of 8-12 repetitions each. But don't overdo it. If you can do only a single set or 3-4 repetitions, do only that at the beginning. Your strength will increase over time, and you will be able to do the required number of sets. Until then, just be patient! Another tip I would like to give you is that before you do weighted exercises with dumbbells and other weights at the gym, try doing them at home using soup cans or water bottles. This is particularly helpful when you don't have access to 1 or 2 lb weights or if you don't want to go to the gym without any idea on how to use weights.

Another important thing to remember is to pay attention to tempo. No, it's not dancing, folks! Tempo simply means rhythm. Any movements that stretch your muscles should be done in a rhythmic manner, so that each time the fibers extend and contract to the same length, dispersing the force in an even manner throughout the muscle. Controlling tempo also controls your movements. You are forced to move in a slow, steady manner rather than relying on momentum to complete an exercise. Real-life exercise is nothing like what you see on commercials; you are not supposed to do 15 sets in under a minute. There is no gain in that, except perhaps torn muscle. What you want to do is take it nice and slow, all the while keeping a rhythm. For example, count to four while lifting a dumbbell, hold for two, then count to four while lowering it to the starting position. You don't have to keep counting, of course! You will become accustomed to the pace soon enough. If you are having problems, use headphones. Play a slow-beat song and move to the beats!

One last thing to know about before we move on to the actual exercises. How do you determine what weights you use? It can be very confusing to someone who is completely new to weighted exercises. A rule of thumb, start with the smallest weights and work your way up. Choose a smaller-sized dumbbell or weight and work with it. You should be able to do 8-12 repetitions comfortably. After that, the muscles of your arms or legs should start to feel tired. Take a break then and let your muscles' cells replenish their oxygen storage and go again. If you must bend backward or if you can't lift the weight slowly, it's too heavy! You should never use momentum/ sudden movements to lift a weight. I know pro weightlifters do that, but there is a special technique to doing that safely. A small mistake could lead to a broken hip. Before you know it, you are getting months of bed rest and constant bad TV instead of getting fit.

So, always be careful with weights. In fact, I would recommend doing many of the following exercises with just your body weight when you're starting out. Test them out and when you are confident enough, start with small weights! You don't have to do all of them, but I recommend trying at least two every week. Don't worry, you got this!!

21 Weighted Exercises

1. Overhead Press (standing or sitting)

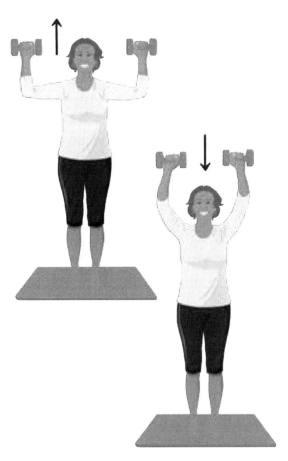

DIRECTIONS

1. Stand or sit upright with your back straight. Keep your hands up, elbows bent, and your forearms against your shoulders/beside your ears.

2. Hold a weight or a dumbbell in each hand at shoulder height. The dumbbells will be above, and your hands will hold them from below, with an overhand grip (thumbs on the inside and knuckles face up).

3. Raise the weights above your head in a controlled upward motion, don't rotate your hands. Use your elbow for strength, and keep pushing it up.

4. Pause briefly at the top, inhale, and return dumbbells to shoulders.

2. Shoulder Squat

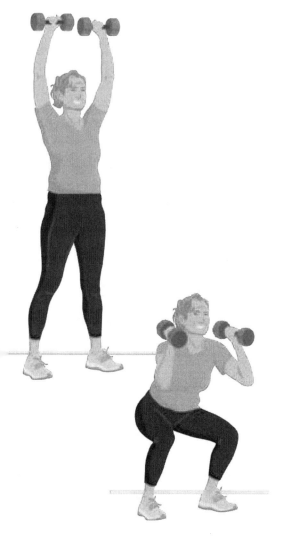

DIRECTIONS

1. Take a dumbbell in each hand.

2. Grip it in your hands so your palms are resting below the dumbbell, and raise your hands to your shoulder, keeping your feet hip-width apart.

3. Brace your abdominals and stand straight with your shoulders pulled back.

4. Lower your body by bending at the knees. Descend until your thighs are parallel to the floor or as far as you can go while maintaining good form (head and back straight, not leaning forward or arched).

5. Hold for a second or two, then press into your heels to straighten your knees and hips and return to a standing position. Use your thighs and abdominals for strength. Your back should stay straight for the duration of the move.

3. Chest Press

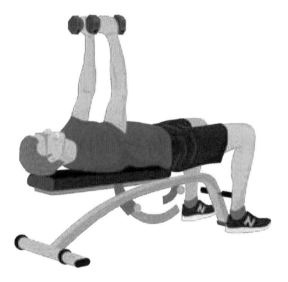

DIRECTIONS

1. Lie on a bench or step and hold dumbbells up over your chest, arms extended (be sure you aren't locking your elbows).

2. Bend the elbows and lower the weights until your elbows are at about 90-degree angles. Your elbows should be at your head level while lying, and the dumbbells should be above your head.

3. Press the weights back up and repeat. Make sure you are not lowering your hands too much.

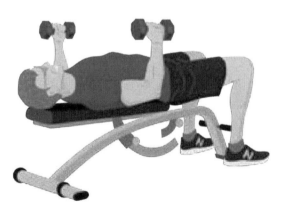

4. Front Raise

1. Stand with your feet shoulder-width apart and hold one dumbbell in each hand. Keep your hands on your side.

2. Lift your arms forward in front of you with the dumbbells. Hold the dumbbells in a way so that the palms should be facing the thighs and the dumbbell is below your palms.

3. Try lifting one hand at a time at first and make a 90-degree angle with your lower body and arms.

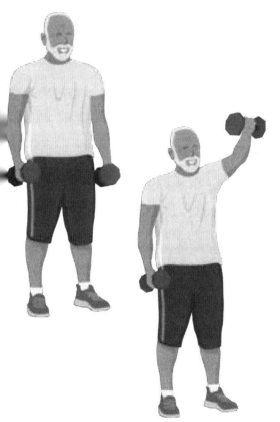

4. While lifting the weights upward, inhale. Keep your arm extended with a slight bend in the elbows and your palms facing down.

5. Pause briefly when your lifted arm is horizontal to the floor, then lower the dumbbells back to your thighs while exhaling.

6. Now do the other arm. After doing that a few times, you can try lifting both hands at once.

Straighten your back and engage your abdominals. Don't bend backward.

5. Arm Curl

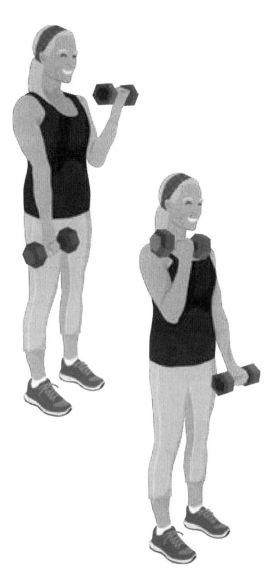

1. Stand tall with your feet about hip-width apart, engaging your abdominals.

2. Hold one dumbbell in each hand, and let your arms relax down at the sides of your body with your palms facing forward.

3. Keeping your upper arms still and shoulders relaxed, bend one arm at the elbow and lift the dumbbell toward your shoulders. Exhale while lifting.

4. Lower the weight to the starting position, then repeat with the opposite arm. Your elbows should stay tucked in close to your ribs while you are doing this exercise.

You can do this both standing and sitting.

6. Bent-over Rows

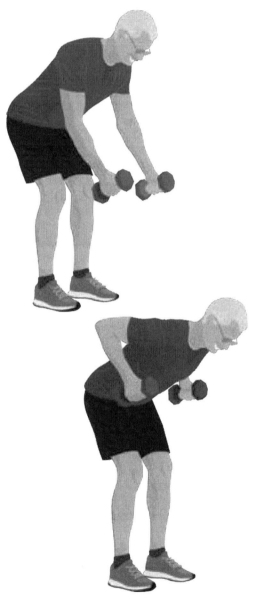

DIRECTIONS

1. Stand with your knees slightly bent and your legs apart.

2. Bend forward at a 45-degree angle and take a deep breath in.

3. Put your weight on your knees and feet. Plant your feet securely on the ground. Hold one dumbbell with each of your hands so that your palms face your body.

4. Standing in that leaned forward position, pull the dumbbells straight up, toward your chest, on an exhale. Make sure your wrists are locked in position as much as possible and take strength from your abdominals while pulling the dumbbells. When lifting the dumbbell up, your upper arms should go no high- er than parallel with your shoulders.

5. Lower the weights in a controlled manner to the starting position as you inhale. Stay bent over until all reps have been completed.

7. Triceps Extension

1. Lie on your back on a gym bench or any flat surface where you can fit your entire body, except your lower legs. Keep your feet flat on the floor so that your knee is bent at 90 degrees with your body.

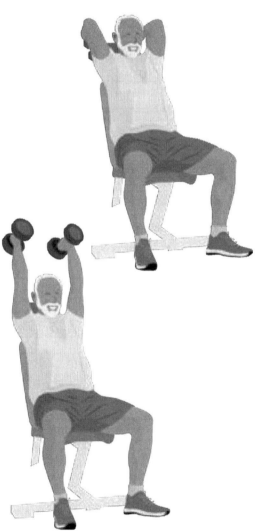

2. Put your arms above you, reach for the ceiling and hold a dumbbell with both of your hands. Your arms holding the dumbbell will be above your chest and abdomen. So, make sure to hold it in a secure grip.

3. Bend your elbows and lower the weight slowly downward and upward toward the back of your head while keeping your arms in the same position and bending your elbows a little.

4. Continue lowering the weight behind your head until the bottom of the dumbbell head is in line with the bench's top.

5. Reverse the movement until the weight is back above your chest. Don't lock your elbows when performing this move and always have someone near you. If your hands suddenly give up, the dumbbell could fall on you and do severe damage.

8. One-arm Row

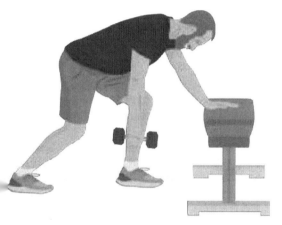

DIRECTIONS

1. Stand beside a platform or bench.

2. Place your left knee on a bench or platform and rest your left hand or forearm on the same platform. So, now you are in a leaning position. Keep your back flat and your abdominals engaged.

3. Hold a weight in your right hand and keep your hands straight down without any wrist rotation. Your hand position should be as if you are hanging the weight down toward the floor with your hand.

4. Bend the elbow and pull the weight straight up in a rowing motion until it's level with your torso or just above it.

5. Keep the weight up there for a few seconds, then lower the weight slowly back down.

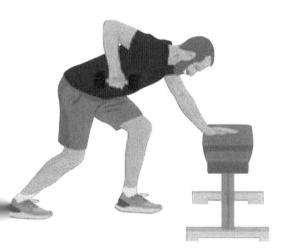

9. Dumbbell Squat to Overhead Press

1. Perform an overhead press as normal.

2. When you lower the dumbbells to your shoulders, bend your knees and sit into a squat.

3. Hold the position for a few seconds and get back up to a standing position.

4. Complete the move by lifting the dumbbells back up to shoulder level.

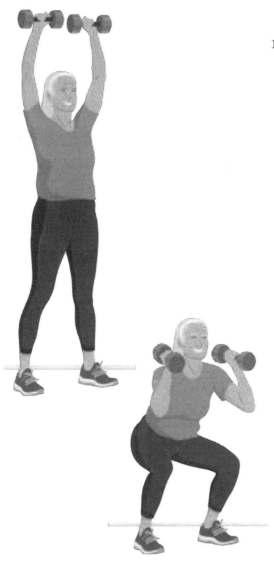

10. Kickback

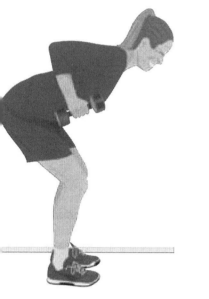

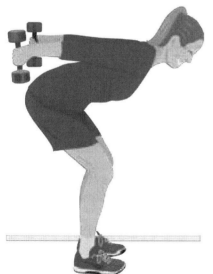

DIRECTIONS

1. Stand straight.

2. Bend at the waist and lean forward. Keep your back flat and abdominals engaged.

3. Keeping this position, take a dumbbell in each hand. Bend your elbow, pull your forearms forward, and put the dumbbells on the side of your chest (your elbows will be raised above your back).

4. Straighten your arms slowly while your upper arms stay in place so that the dumbbells go backward (above your back).

5. Lower the dumbbells and repeat.

You can make this move with one arm or both arms. Make sure to bend your knees and keep your core engaged.

11. Deadlift

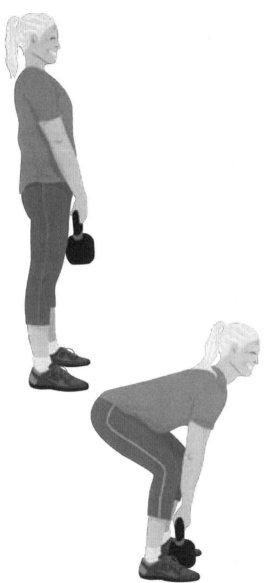

DIRECTIONS

1. Stand straight with your fee shoulder length apart.

2. Hold one dumbbell in each hand i front of you, at thigh level.

3. Lean forward, bend from the wais about 45 degrees, and lower th weights toward the floor with you back straight and shoulders locked

4. Return to start and repeat.

You need to keep your shoulders back while pulling the weight up and down. Caving in the shoulder will lead to rounding and hurting your back.

12. Resistance Band: One arm Chest Press

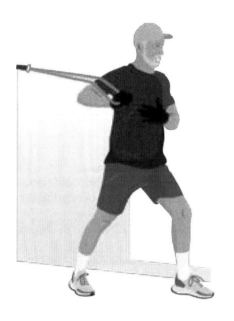

DIRECTIONS

1. Stand straight and wrap the band around one of your hands. The other end should be tied to a sturdy object behind you.

2. Hold the band with your left hand and step forward, away from the sturdy object, until you can feel tension on the band.

3. Then take one step forward and keep your left arm back.

4. Lift and bend your left arm at the elbow, with the band coming under the arm and the elbow bent at 90 degrees, palm facing inward, grip the band and move your left arm forward.

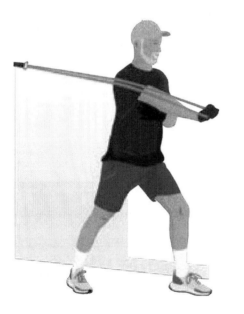

Put your right arm against your body while doing this and take strength from your chest and shoulder muscles.

13. Resistance Band: Lat Pulls

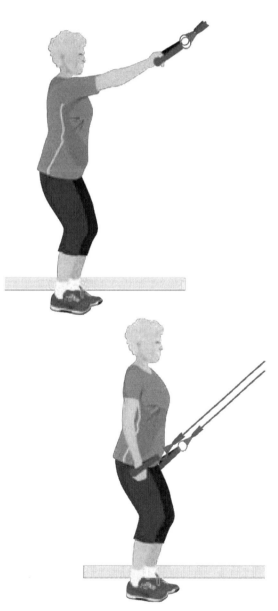

DIRECTIONS

1. Attach the middle of the band to a hook on the wall.

2. Hold one end of the band in each hand and sit at enough distance so your hands are above your head (sitting) or forward (standing).

3. Pull the ends of the band downward toward your legs.

4. Pull down until your hands are completely down and your palms are against your thighs. Then, go back to the original position slowly.

*Stand or sit straight for this exercise.

14. Squat Curl Knee Lift

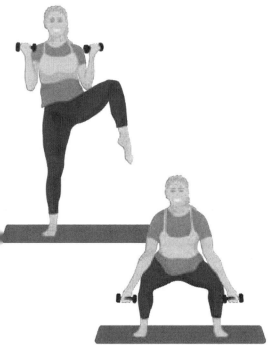

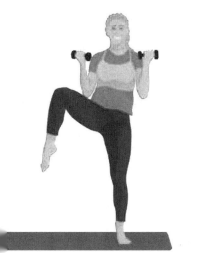

DIRECTIONS

1. Start in a squat position with your weight on your heels and your arms hanging at your sides, dumbbells in hand.

2. Use your lower back muscles to press up.

3. Stand up while lifting your right knee as you curl the weights to your shoulders.

4. Slowly lower the weights back down and return to a squat position. Repeat with the left knee.

You need good balance to do this exercise, so if you feel unsteady, skip this one. Alternatively, you can try doing it next to a wall or chair.

15. Dumbbell Scaption

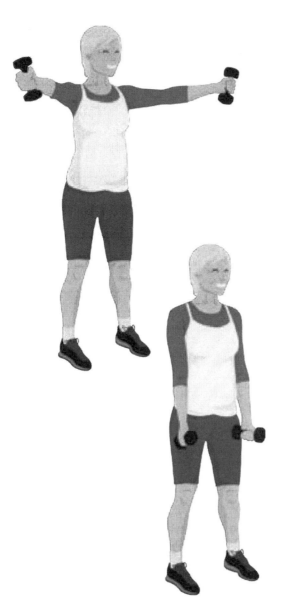

DIRECTIONS

1. Stand straight with one dumbbell in each hand. Keep your arms straight at your sides so that the palms are facing inwards.

2. Take strength from your abdominals and core while lifting the dumbbells up. Keep your hands straight.

3. Pull the dumbbells at a 45-degree angle with your body.

4. Raise the weights slowly above your shoulders and then to your head level, wait for a few seconds, then slowly lower your arms.

16. Stability Ball: Side Leg Lift

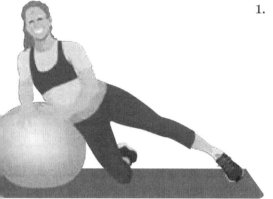

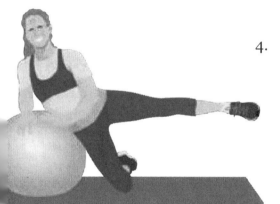

DIRECTIONS

1. Kneel on your right knee with the ball to your right side.

2. Slightly lean with your right side on the ball and use your right arm to hold the ball to your sides. Keep your left leg straightened out to the side while the right leg is bent on the floor.

3. Slowly lift your left leg, and then lower it. It should take about 6 seconds to lift and 6 seconds to lower it.

4. Switch sides once you've completed one side.

You can do this exercise by both kneeling and keeping your legs straight. Above, I have given you directions to start with the easier one kneeling.

17. Goblet Squat

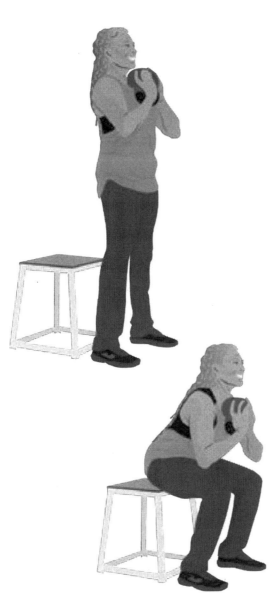

1. Stand straight with your feet wide. They should be placed more than shoulder-length apart.

2. Hold a dumbbell with each hand midlevel to your chest.

3. Using your thighs for strength, move down and position yourself into a squat. You need to keep your shoulders and your back straight.

4. Raise back up slowly without leaning forward. Keep the dumbbell in front of you at all times.

18. Dumbbell Bench Press

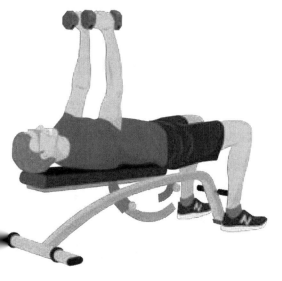

DIRECTIONS

1. Lie on your back on a flat bench.

2. Hold two dumbbells, one in each hand, in an overhand grip. Keep them at your chest level or above your chest.

3. Push up slowly until your arms are straight, hold for a few seconds.

4. Lower slowly.

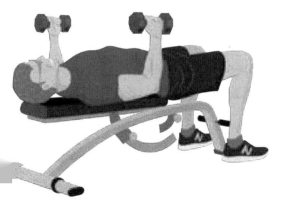

19. Crossbody Hammer Curl

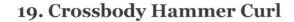

DIRECTIONS

1. Stand straight with your back straight and your feet apart slightly with one dumbbell in each hand.

2. Pull your right hand up toward your left shoulder and chest.

3. Straighten your hand and return to the original position.

4. Repeat on the other side.

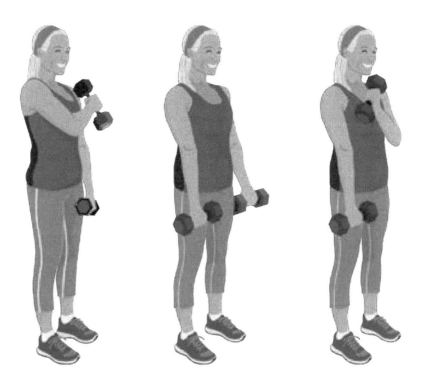

20. Single Dumbbell Shoulder Raise

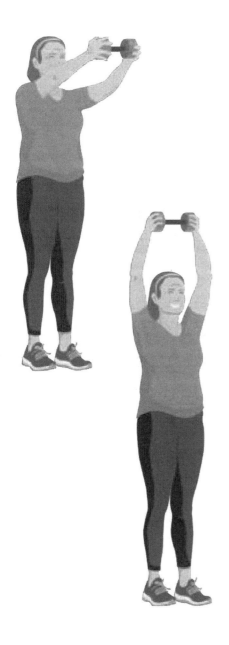

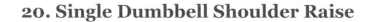

DIRECTIONS

1. Put one hand on either side of a dumbbell and hold it between your legs.

2. Holding both ends of the dumbbell, slowly lift it upward and backwards above your head.

3. Hold for a few seconds, then slowly lower it down and repeat.

21. Forward Lunge

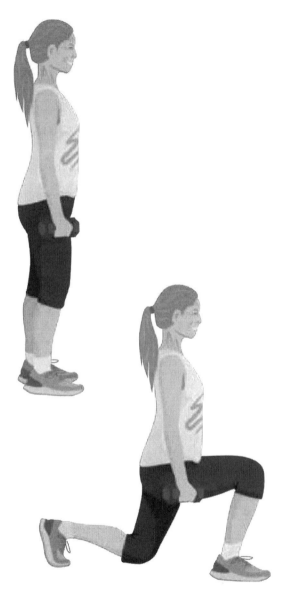

1. Stand up straight with a dumbbell in each hand, arms hanging at your sides. Your palms should face your thighs, and your feet should be a little less than shoulder-width apart.

2. Inhale and take a big step forward with your right leg. Put your right foot firmly on the ground.

3. Bend both knees and put the left knee on the floor keeping the right thigh nearly parallel to the ground, but don't let the right knee go past the tip of your toes. The left leg is balanced on the toes.

4. Step the right foot back on an exhale to return to the starting position and repeat with the left leg.

This move requires good balance, so if you struggle with that, start by doing the exercise without weights.

Chapter 8: Exercise Modifications: Obesity

"Take care of your body. It's the only place you have to live"

Jim Rohn

Most people embark upon their exercise journeys to get slimmer and fitter. However, when getting into an exercise routine, it's important to have a realistic approach to your fitness. Having a goal in mind is not a bad thing. Yet, if you are expecting too much in too short a time, it will be very easy for you to give up. Any changes you do manage to make through workouts will fall short, and you won't be able to enjoy your new habits.

Let's face it, it's unreasonable to expect you to start running marathons or doing deadlifts after only a month or two of exercising. Particularly if you are out of practice or haven't lifted excess weight for a long time. For people who weigh more than average, it's even harder. Because they carry their own weight when they do any kind of movement, it takes more effort. Running, for example, becomes more difficult the more you weigh. However, that is only more reason to exercise; so that simple movements become easier for you. There are plenty of workouts an obese person can do efficiently without becoming too quickly exhausted. In this chapter, we're going to look at some exercises that can be performed regardless of weight and mobility.

We will focus on smart and effective compound exercises. These will ensure that you're making progress and building up your strength, even if they seem easier than other workout routines. As you do these exercises more regularly, your confidence and comfort with exercise will continue to grow. Also, most of the exercises mentioned here are based on basic movement patterns that you use in your day-to-day life, such as sitting, standing, reaching, and lifting. So, as you go through your routine, you will see improvements in your daily life as well.

Warm-ups

Each day before you start exercising, make sure you allot at least 10 minutes for warm-up. Two to three minutes of walking or calisthenics will raise your body temperature and warm up your muscles without causing too much fatigue at the beginning of the workout. (Calisthenics are exercises that only use your weight.)

To make things easier, start with standing stretches rather than stretches that require you to get up and down off the floor. Standing exercises are easier to do. Plus, they increase the mobility of your upper body, which we need most in our daily lives. Here are some stretches to start with:

Gastrocnemius Stretch

Gastrocnemius stretch sounds difficult but is very easy to do.

1. All you need to do is stand up straight, facing the wall.

2. Put your hands forward and on the wall and bend your right knee.

3. Lean forward while keeping your left leg straight and stretched behind (your heels should be placed on the floor). You will feel your calves stretching.

Standing Soleus Stretch

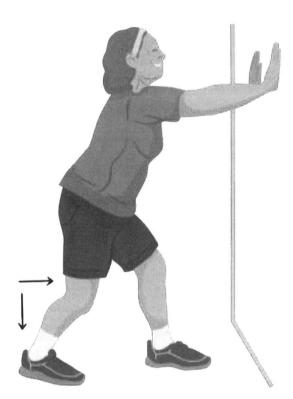

DIRECTIONS

1. Position yourself in front of the wall, closer than before, and put your hand's palm first on the wall.

2. Take a step back with your left leg and start bending your right knee while moving the left leg backwards.

3. Bend the knee to about 110-90 degrees and stop.

Keep both heels firmly on the ground while doing this.

Standing Latissimus Dorsi Stretch

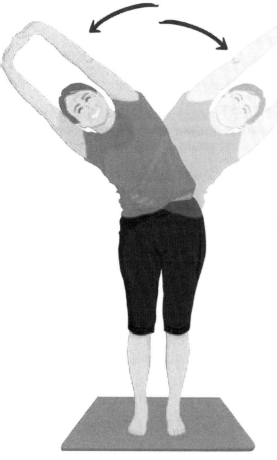

DIRECTIONS

1. Start by standing straight up with your hands beside your body.

2. Lift your hands above your head.

3. Lean-to one side while keeping your hands up above your head. Lean-to the side as much as you can. You need to keep facing the wall while doing this.

4. Slowly get back to standing straight and proceed to lean toward the other side.

126

Exercises

After warming up properly, you can move on to exercising. Here are some simple moves to try out:

Chair Sit to Stand

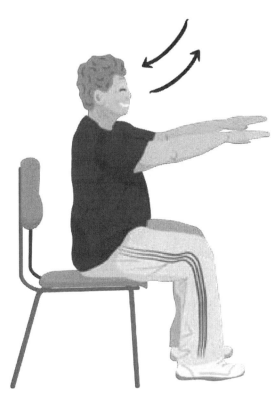

DIRECTIONS

1. Sit straight on a bench with your back straight.

2. Pull up your arms and position them in front of your body.

3. Stand up with your hands straight ahead by taking strength from your thighs.

4. Keep your body in an upright standing position for a few seconds, then slowly return to the initial seated position.

You will not be getting the full depth of a squat in this exercise as you are using the bench. However, the goal of this workout is to get your muscles used to the up and down motion. You can increase the difficulty of the exercise as you become more comfortable with it.

Box Squats

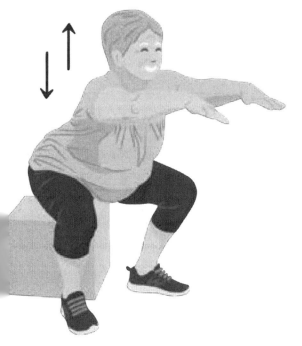

DIRECTIONS

1. Stand in front of a cardboard box or bench with your arms straight in front of you.

2. Bend your knees and sit down to a squat. Keep your back straight and your shoulders back until you are almost sitting on the surface of the seat—like sitting on an invisible chair.

3. Push back up, taking strength from your thighs and keeping your feet firmly on the ground.

4. Return to a standing position.

This varies from the sit and stands because you are never placing your full weight on the bench. Of course, if you start to feel off-balance, go ahead and sit. You can try again when you feel recovered.

High Knee Walks

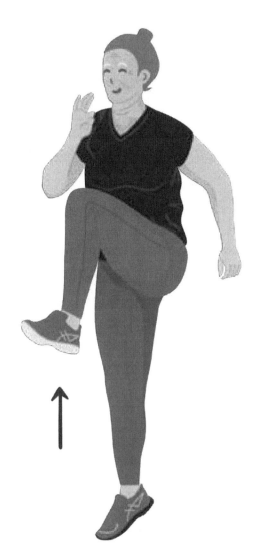

1. Stand straight. Start with your arms straight at your side.

2. Put your arms up and bend your elbows with your forearms at the side of your chest. Put your feet shoulder-width apart and plant your feet firmly on the ground.

3. Raise your left knee toward your chest as high as you can while standing straight.

4. Put it back down slowly and step forward as you do so.

5. Repeat with the right knee, and walk forward like this.

Step-ups

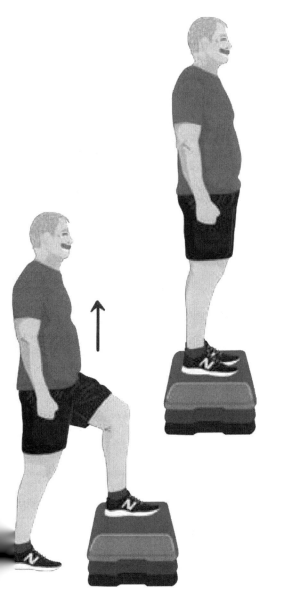

DIRECTIONS

1. Stand in front of the stairs of your house (or find a surface high enough to reach shin to knee height).

2. Slowly place your right foot on the first step and push on with your right foot to lift your left, placing your left foot beside it.

3. Bend your right knee and step back down with the left foot.

4. Bring the right foot down to meet the left foot on the ground.

5. Repeat on the other leg.

Don't use too high or too low steps, or you may lose your balance.

Core Exercises

Farmer's Walk

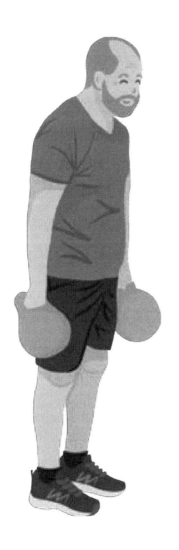

1. Start with light weights and place them on the floor on either side of your body.

2. Lean forward and reach down, bend at the hips and knees, and lift the weights up by holding one in each arm. When you are lifting them up, take strength by extending your hips and knees.

3. Hold the weights at your side and stand tall, keeping shoulders, back, and core engaged.

4. Walk forward at an even pace until you've completed a predetermined number of steps.

5. After you have completed a set or you are tired, place the weights down slowly by only bending your knee but not leaning down or bending your elbow.

For the duration of the exercise, keep a tight core and neutral spine.

Standing Wall Plank

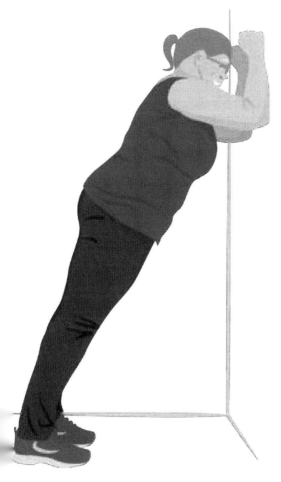

DIRECTIONS

1. Stand tall while keeping a straight back.

2. Put your palms on the wall firmly. Lean on your elbows and lower arms against the wall. Your forearms should be against the wall.

3. Keep your shoulders straight and back, lean forward, and put your weight on your forearms for 30 seconds or as long as possible.

4. Step out and back up.

Russian Twist

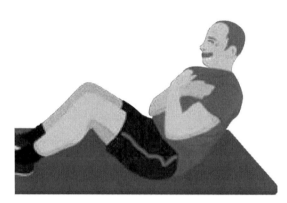

1. Sit straight, put your legs stretched in front of you and keep your knees bent. Do it while keeping your heels on the floor.

2. Lean back and balance your weight on your hips.

3. Slightly raise your legs (keep them together). A few inches are enough. Keep your knees slightly bent.

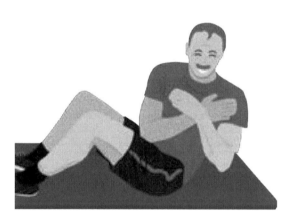

4. Put your arms on your chest by bending at the elbow.

5. Twist your body side to side by twisting your torso and legs in the opposite directions. Your torso and legs should move with your hips as the center point. When moving your torso, move both of your arms in the same direction. With your eyes follow the movement of your hands.

If keeping your legs in the air is difficult, keep your heels touching the ground initially. You will soon get used to the movement.

Dead Bug

A dead bug is an easy core exercise to do, especially if your waist is larger.

DIRECTIONS

1. To start, lie on your back with your face up.

2. Put your arms up; raise them toward the ceiling.

3. Keep one leg (right) stretched straight and raise the other one (left). Bend your left knee so that your thighs are perpendicular to the floor and your calf and feet are horizontal to the floor.

4. Put one hand (left) up beside your head and keep the other (right) pointed up.

5. Alternate the positions of right and left hand and right and left legs.

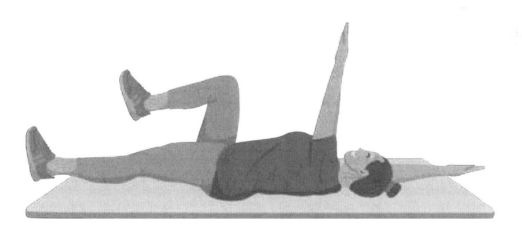

Low impact cardio

Low-impact cardio is the type of exercise where there is an increase in heart rate without putting too much stress on your body. Any form of low-impact cardio will help you burn a decent number of calories while reducing the risk of potential injury.

These exercises can be easily adapted to your schedule. One simple way is to incorporate fast walking, swimming, cycling, the elliptical, etc., into your routine for an easy way to start shedding the pounds. The faster you do these exercises, the more calories you burn. You may not be able to keep the pace for long, but that's fine. You'll want to keep your cardio sessions smaller in duration at first as well. Start with 5-minute chunks of exercise and rests of 2-3 minutes in between. You can increase these time frames as you become more comfortable with exercising.

Weight training

Weight training is not necessarily a must when you are trying to lose weight. The primary goal of exercising for weight loss is to increase the number of calories spent. It should be much more than the daily calorie intake. Weight training does burn a lot of calories, so in that sense, you can do some weights. Many weight training exercises are designed to be bodyweight exercises (using only your body and no extra weights), but there's no reason that weight training needs to be off-limits. When done correctly and in a controlled manner, it is a safer option than jumping or skipping for many.

Diet

Diet is the unseen part of weight loss, even when you are losing weight through exercising. If your diet is not changed, no matter how hard you work, you won't see much change. In fact, you may end up getting heavier!

There are a variety of foods you can eat when you are exercising. A common and acceptable technique that tends to work is a diet heavily enriched with fruits and berries. Being natural products, fruits and berries usually have you covered in terms of the vitamins and minerals necessary for healthy joints and muscles. Individuals over the age of 60 should always consider starting their day with some fruit. Fruit will give you the sweet taste without the negative consequences of processed sugar, and it will boost your immune system, cardiac health, and metabolism. Colorful fruits and veggies are especially beneficial. Most of them contain carotene and retinoids—the activated form of vitamin A that slows down aging. They also contain a lot of vitamin C. This is something that speeds up healing, improve the blood supply, and makes joints and cartilage strong. I know most of us to feel like it's too late for the healthy stuff, but it's not. Fresh fruits, fish, some meat (yes, meat can be healthy too), and lots of veggies will bring about a faster change in your metabolism when combined with exercise. Even if you are moderately healthy and have no problem aside from weight, a nutritious, well-rounded diet is a must. It not only helps you reduce weight but also keeps your mind healthy. Research proves that a well-rounded diet, like the Mediterranean diet, helps prevent depression in older adults (Skarupski et al., 2013).

That being said, please don't start drinking horrible smelling smoothies for breakfast and eating cardboard-like veggies for lunch. No good comes from force-feeding yourself unappetizing food in the name of health. It is actually proven that for healthy aging, food satisfaction is equally important as a nutritious meal. Food can be both healthy and tasty!

References:

Skarupski, K. A., Tangney, C. C., Li, H., Evans, D. A., & Morris, M. C. (2013). Mediterranean diet and depressive symptoms among older adults over time. The Journal of nutrition, health & aging, 17(5), 441-445.

Chapter 9: Exercise Modifications: Arthritis

> *"Use it or lose it"*
> Jimmy Conners

Although arthritis is a disease where mobility is restricted, exercise is beneficial for reducing its symptoms. Arthritis is an autoimmune disease. This means your own body's defense cells are attacking your body, namely the cells of your joints. This leads to limitation of movement and pain. However when you exercise, the movements improve joint mobility and lessen the pain somewhat. It also increases strength, flexibility, reduces joint pain, and combats fatigue. However, the thought of exercising when you're already in pain can be daunting. Thankfully, even moderate exercise can help reduce your symptoms and keep you moving.

How Exercise Helps

Arthritis patients suffer from inflamed joints, which leads to pain and disability. Exercising improves blood flow to the joint, and as a result, the synovial fluid (fluid inside the joint) flow is increased. Thai Chi helps in reducing inflammation which is the source of the pain. A clinical research study based on 64 patients with RA and an average age of 60 showed that short-term programs of intensive exercises are well tolerated by patients with active arthritis (Van den Ende et al.

2000)[1]. Furthermore, the results of the study also showed that patients in the intensive exercise program showed a statistically significant improvement of muscle strength after completion and after six months of follow-up.

According to research, patients also suffer from muscle loss due to loss of movement. A paper published in the Journal of Aging Research mentions, "Most RA patients suffer from an accelerated loss of muscle mass, a condition known as 'rheumatoid cachexia.' This loss contributes to disability and has a significant impact on an individuals' quality of life." According to the same research, "High-intensity resistance exercise has been shown to safely reverse cachexia in patients with RA and, as a consequence of this restoration of muscle mass, to substantially improve physical function and reduce disability in RA patients" (Cooney et al., 2011)[2].

Exercises for the Arthritis Patient

Range of Motion Exercises

These exercises will relieve stiffness and increase your ability to move your joints through a full range of motion.

- raising your arms over your head and reaching toward the sky
- rolling your shoulders forward and backward
- head tilts, forward and back
- wrist bends
- finger bends and finger spreads
- toe curls
- plantar flexion
- ankle circles
- ball kicks

- leg raises
- glute kicks
- cross-body leg raises
- arm kickbacks
- arm circles
- weightless bicep curls

Strengthening Exercises

- Low-Intensity Yoga
- Leg lifts
- Leg extension
- Hip bridges
- Wall squats

Aerobic Exercises

Low-impact aerobic exercises such as walking, biking, swimming, and using the elliptical are great for arthritis. The goal with aerobic exercise is to find an activity that you can enjoy and can complete consistently—most days of the week. I would recommend a morning run or jogging, as the symptoms are usually worse in the morning.

Tips to Protect Your Joints

- **Keep the impact low and move gently.** You'll want to begin with range of motion exercise to help warm up your joints before moving on t strength or aerobic exercise.

- **Apply heat.** Heat can relax your joints and muscles and relieve pain as it increases blood supply. Use a warm towel, hot pack, or shower, and apply for about 20 minutes (the treatments should be warm, not uncomfortably hot)

- **Go slowly.** Your movements should always be slow, precise, and controlled—never painful. If you notice swelling or redness in your joints, slow down and rest for a day or two.

- **Ice afterward.** Apply ice to your joints for up to 20 minutes after activity, particularly if that activity causes joint swelling. Ice reduces swelling pretty fast. You can also apply topical NSAIDs like ibuprofen for fast pain relief. But only occasionally and with doctors' consent.

References:

1. Van den Ende, C. H. M., Breedveld, F. C., Le Cessie, S., Dijkmans, B. A. C., De Mug, A. W., & Hazes, J. M. W. (2000). Effect of intensive exercise on patients with active rheumatoid arthritis: a randomised clinical trial. Annals of the rheumatic diseases, 59(8), 615-621.

2. Cooney, J. K., Law, R. J., Matschke, V., Lemmey, A. B., Moore, J. P., Ahmad, Z., ... & Thom, J. M. (2011). Benefits of exercise in rheumatoid arthritis. Journal of aging research, 2011.

Chapter 10: Exercise Modifications: Bad Knees

It's likely that you've experienced discomfort in your knees while attempting to move a large object. Maybe you've avoided lifting anything at all because you're afraid of injuring your knees. Your fear is well-founded. Knees bear the brunt of your weight and are responsible for a large portion of your mobility therefore, taking good care of them is a good idea. They also have a lot of moving parts, such as ligaments and cartilage, as well as muscles and bones. These can be harmed by injury or natural wear and tear, making it challenging to stay active and participate in physical activities. Luckily, there are techniques to defy time and delay or even avoid knee troubles. For example, land-based therapeutic exercises are shown to have excellent results for an osteoarthritic knee. Results accumulated from several research articles support this theory. Among these trials, "44 indicated that exercise significantly reduced pain and improved physical function to a moderate degree immediately after treatment while evidence from 13 studies revealed that exercise significantly improved quality of life immediately after treatment with small effect."[1]

Fortunately, most of the exercises we will do fall into this category. They can help maintain your knees' fitness and allow you to walk a mile longer or lift heavier weights without risking injury. In this chapter, we'll walk you through exercises that help age-proof your knees.

Stretches

Lower body stretching exercises, according to the American Academy of Orthopedic Surgeons, can assist and boost the range of motion and elasticity in your kneecap. This can help you move your knee more easily, without losing much energy. Warm up for at least 5 to 10 minutes before beginning your stretching routine. Warming up with low-impact sports like stationary cycling, walking, or utilizing an elliptical machine is an excellent idea. Do the following three stretches once you've warmed up. Then, repeat after you've finished the knee strengthening exercises.

Hamstring Stretch

Stretching enhances your range of motion and how far your joints can move in different directions and keeps you flexible. It also aids in the prevention of pain and injury.

DIRECTIONS

1. Warm up for at least 5 minutes.

2. When you're ready to stretch your hamstrings, lie down.

3. Wrap your right foot in a bedsheet.

4. Pull the leg up with the help of the sheet and keep it straight.

5. Hold for 20 seconds before lowering your leg.

6. Repeat the process twice more. After that, switch legs.

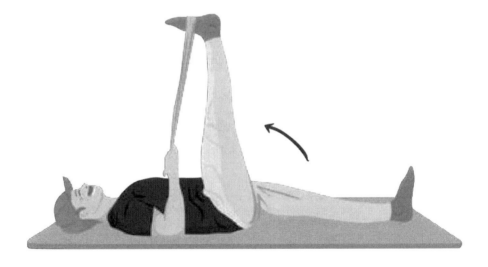

Calf Stretch

This stretch focuses on the lower leg muscles, particularly the calf muscles.

DIRECTIONS

1. For balance, grab a chair and bend your right leg.

2. Step back with your left leg and straighten it slowly, pressing your left heel to the floor.

3. Hold for 20 seconds, then swap legs.

4. Lean forward and bend your right knee deeper, but not past your toes, for a deeper stretch.

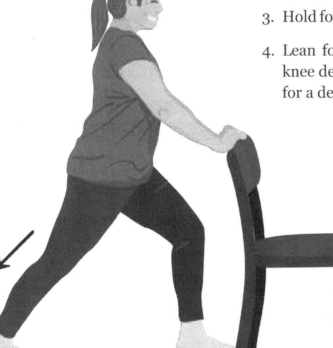

Strength

Hamstring Curls

The lying hamstring curl predominantly targets the hamstrings, which is evident from its name. The hamstring is made up of three muscles in the back of your leg: the biceps femoris, the semitendinosus, and semimembranosus. You should feel a profound tension in these muscles during this exercise. Rest assured, the tension is worth it because it is an excellent exercise for hamstring growth and strength. This exercise will not only improve your lower-body strength but will also help you avoid injury and improve your performance in other exercises.

DIRECTIONS

1. Lie flat on your stomach and slowly bring your feet as close to your rear as possible.

2. Hold for 30 seconds or as long as it is comfortable.

3. Do three sets of 15 repetitions.

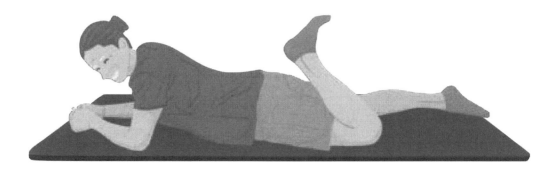

Straight Leg Raise

Straight leg raises are a terrific option if you want a knee exercise that won't strain your leg muscles. This basic activity strengthens the quadriceps and hamstrings, which help the knees move freely.

DIRECTIONS

1. Lie down on your back on the floor with your legs straight out in front of you.

2. Raise one leg toward the ceiling, keeping the other flat on the floor in front of your buttocks. This is the leg that will be supporting you.

3. Raise your opposite leg as high as you can while keeping it straight out to align with your opposing supporting knee. Your muscles will be working to lift it.

4. Return your straight leg to the ground.

5. Repeat 10 times more and switch legs. Complete up to three sets.

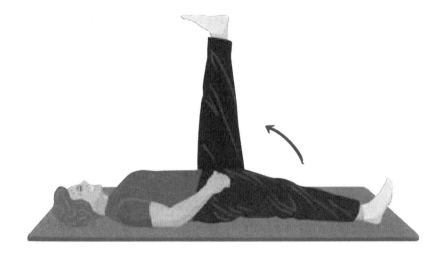

Quad Sets

Is the straight leg raise too difficult for you? If so, you can try quad sets instead. You don't have to raise your leg with these. Simply tighten one leg's thigh muscles, commonly known as quads, at a time. [2]

DIRECTIONS

1. Lie down on the floor.

2. Maintain a relaxed posture with both legs on the ground.

3. For 5 seconds, flex and hold your left leg tense.

4. Relax.

5. Perform two sets of ten repetitions each. After each set, switch legs.

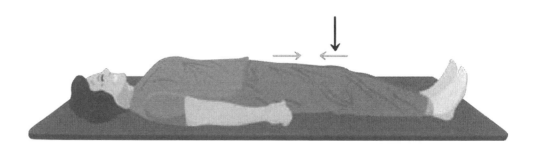

Seated Hip March

This one will help you strengthen your hips and thighs, which will assist with everyday activities such as walking and standing up.

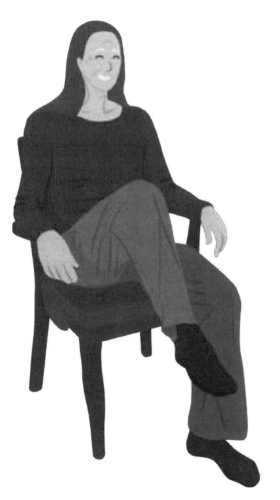

DIRECTIONS

1. In a chair, sit up straight.

2. Keep your toes on the floor and kick your left foot back slightly.

3. Raise your right foot off the ground with your knee bent.

4. Hold your right leg up in the air for three seconds.

5. Lower your foot to the ground slowly.

6. Perform two sets of ten repetitions each. After each set, switch legs.

Modification: Is it too difficult? Lift your leg with the help of your hands.

Pillow Squeeze

This exercise strengthens the inside of your legs, which aids with knee suppor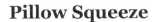

1. Lie down on your back with your knees bent.

2. Between the knees, place a pillow.

3. Squeeze your knees together and squash the pillow in the space between them.

4. Hold the position for 5 seconds.

5. Relax your legs.

6. Perform two sets of ten repetitions each. After each set, switch legs.

Modification: If you find it difficult to do this exercise lying down, you'll be glad to know that this exercise can also be done while seated!

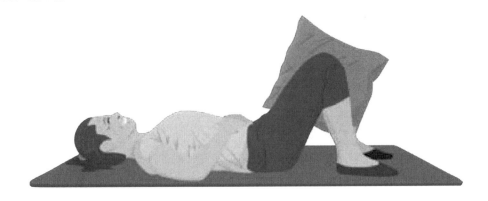

Heel Raise

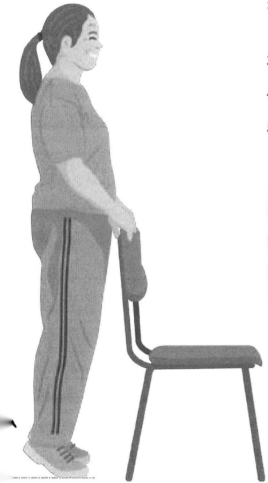

DIRECTIONS

1. Stand tall and support yourself on the back of a chair.

2. Raise your toes off the ground and lift your heels off the ground.

3. Hold the position for 3 seconds.

4. Lower both heels to the ground slowly.

5. Perform two sets of ten repetitions each.

Modification: Sit in a chair and perform the same activity if you find it too challenging.

150

Side Leg Raise

DIRECTIONS

1. For steadiness, stand and grip the back of a chair.

2. Your weight should be on your left leg.

3. Keep the right leg straight and the outer leg muscles stiff as you stand tall and lift the right leg out to the side.

4. Hold for 3 seconds before lowering the leg slowly. Perform two sets of ten repetitions each. After each set, switch legs.

If it feels difficult in the beginning, don't worry. Leg height will gradually increase as your body becomes accustomed to the process.

One leg Balance

This technique assists you in bending over or getting into and out of vehicles.

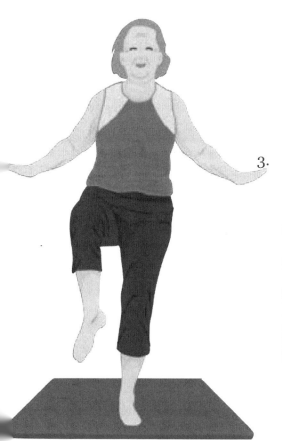

DIRECTIONS

1. Slowly lift one foot off the floor while standing behind your kitchen counter without holding on.

2. The objective is to remain balanced for 20 seconds without touching the counter.

3. Switch sides after making this move twice.

Modification: If you find it too simple, try maintaining your balance for a longer period of time. Alternatively, attempt it blindfolded.

Side Steps

Side steps are simple to take and will enable you to retain your balance and mobility. These may be done almost anywhere and don't require any particular equipment.

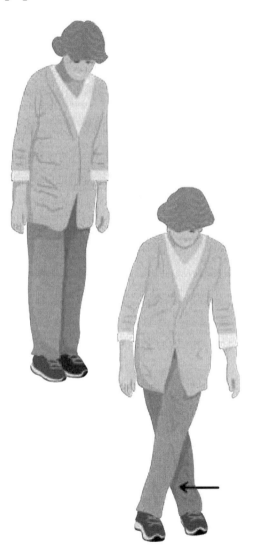

DIRECTIONS

1. Stand with your feet hip-width apart in a neutral position.

2. Take a step to the side with your right leg, widening your legs.

3. Next, bring your left leg up beside your right.

4. Take a step to the side with your left foot. Then, bring your right leg back in.

5. Do 10-12 reps for a total of three sets.

Modification: When doing side steps, add some ankle weights for a more cardiovascular workout.

Knee problems affect many seniors around the world. The most common knee ailments seen in the medical field include tendonitis, osteoarthritis, sprains, and discomfort. Tendonitis is a condition in which the knee joints become inflamed and swollen as a result of overuse or incorrect use. Those with an athletic background are more likely to suffer. Osteoarthritis is the breakdown of cartilage in the bones and joints over time. Osteoarthritis produces weakness, discomfort, and stiffness, as well as the potential for additional injury. Furthermore, weakened joints or muscles are more prone to sprains. Knee sprains are common as people age because their bodies must work harder to handle their weight, despite the fact that their strength is deteriorating. Knee discomfort and degeneration are the most common causes of falls in the elderly. Because the knees bear the weight of so much of the upper body, falls and mishaps are more frequent.

If you're suffering from knee pain as a result of an injury, surgery, or arthritis, mild stretching and strengthening activities can help relieve the discomfort while also improving your flexibility and range of motion. Exercising an injured or arthritic knee may seem paradoxical, yet it is actually better for your knee than sitting idle. If you don't move your knee, it will stiffen. This makes the discomfort greater, and it becomes more difficult to go about your everyday tasks. The muscles that support your knee joint can be strengthened with gentle stretching and strengthening activities. Stronger muscles can help your knee joint move more readily by reducing the impact and tension on it.

Tips

Aside from the exercises mentioned above, here are some useful tips that will help you keep your knees in optimal condition:

Keep a Proper Body Weight.

The pressure on your knees increases with each step you take. Walking necessitates movements from the tendons, ligaments, and muscles. The meniscus, or cartilage in the knee, serves to absorb the impact of each step, stumble, or shock.

Excess body weight puts additional pressure and impact on the knees, as well as the rest of the body. One of the primary causes of physical damage and health decline is being overweight. Additionally, you also need to build some strength if you want to keep exercising. Include strength training in your exercise regime to ensure your body becomes more capable little by little. Strength training, surprisingly, has an extremely beneficial effect on the health of older adults. So, not only you will get stronger with this training, you will also become healthier.[3]

Maintain a Regular Workout Schedule

It's not about how much you can manage when it comes to exercise. It all comes down to being consistent and purposeful with your health. Knee exercises should be incorporated into your daily workout regimen to help them age gracefully with you, avoiding early degradation and injury. Healthy behaviours are essential for general well-being! Make it a habit, just like you would for bathing or brushing your teeth. Aim for 3-5 times a week of exercise.

Steer Clear of Injuries

It's critical to understand what perfect form looks and feels like before beginning any physical training practice. Each movement has a right and wrong way to perform when executing an activity. The wrong approach to a stretch or a strengthening exercise might harm your body. Make sure you have someone to guide you in the appropriate form before beginning new or more strenuous activities to avoid injury.

Don't discount mobility and stretching

Strength is crucial when it comes to knees. It's also critical for maintaining flexibility, balance and relieving the tightness around the knees. Basic stretching and balance exercises should be included with any strength-building goals you have in mind. With all of the effort you put into strengthening your body, you don't want it to become so stiff that it can't move.

You should expect to see effects over time if you execute the correct knee strengthening exercises with good form and consistency. Listen to your body, stretch frequently, and get moving! Keep in mind that good habits lead to a stronger body. Make your workouts enjoyable and seek professional assistance specific to you and any conditions you may be experiencing. You'll be sturdy enough to withstand all of life's challenges for years to come if your knees arestronger.

References:

1. Fransen, M., McConnell, S., Harmer, A. R., Van der Esch, M., Simic, M., & Bennell, K. L. (2015). Exercise for osteoarthritis of the knee. *Cochrane database of systematic reviews*, (1).

2. Hafez, A. R., Al-Johani, A. H., Zakaria, A. R., Al-Ahaideb, A., Buragadda, S., Melam, G. R., & Kachanathu, S. J. (2013). Treatment of knee osteoarthritis in relation to hamstring and quadriceps strength. *Journal of physical therapy science*, 25(11), 1401-1405.

3. Seguin, R., & Nelson, M. E. (2003). The benefits of strength training for older adults. *American journal of preventive medicine*, 25(3), 141-149.

Chapter 11: Exercise Modifications: Heart Conditions

> *"Exercise should be regarded as tribute to the heart."*
> Gene Tunney

Among the diseases that are most prevalent in people our age, diabetes and heart problems are at the top of the list. Having a heart condition even the simple ones like high blood pressure puts restrictions on your movements. You can't really jog or swim as you would like. Anything that gets your heart beating too fast or puts too much pressure on it is a risk. Also, doing exercises is very difficult for people with heart conditions; they get tired easily and usually have less energy. Therefore, despite doctors' advice, many heart patients do not exercise.

When done correctly, exercise can strengthen your heart and allow you to be more active without initiating chest pain or other symptoms. The key here is to accomplish goals little by little until it feels easier. According to research, regular exercise can improve functional capacity and quality of life in several domains (Bocalini et al., 2008)[1]. Not only that, having regular exercise can reverse the damage in cardiac tissue by increasing the blood supply and strengthening both heart and the vessels within. In this chapter, we are going to walk you through three types of exercises that will help you achieve optimal physical fitness even with your heart condition.

Physical activity is an important part of maintaining excellent heart health. It's one of your most powerful methods for strengthening your heart muscle, maintaining a healthy weight, and preventing arterial damage. This damage can be caused by excessive cholesterol, high blood sugar, and high blood pressure, which can lead to a heart attack or stroke. Multiple forms of exercise are required to achieve total fitness. "Exercise of moderate intensity may benefit many elderly persons in numerous and complementary ways (e.g., cardiovascular status, fracture risk, functional ability, and mental processing)," according to Elward K. and E B Larson.[2] These researchers believe that, even for people over 65 with cardiovascular conditions, exercising is safe. In their paper they mentioned, "Exercise in the elderly probably needs to be tailored, and when possible, individualized, with the specific objectives of the person or group in mind. For example, patients with cardiovascular disease benefit from exercises focused on controlled intensity.

However, if you have a cardiac issue, it's strongly recommended that you get medical advice before beginning any fitness regimen.

Preparation

Before beginning any exercise, you should know about the three important phases.

Warm-up: This portion should last approximately 5 minutes. It aids in the preparation of your body for activity, reduces stress on your heart and muscles, and aids in the prevention of sore muscles. Warm up your muscles by marching in place for a few minutes before stretching. You should slowly bend into the required position with each stretching exercise, just going as far as you can without pain. Hold each posture for 30 seconds and repeat each stretch many times throughout the exercise. Always remember to not let your limbs bounce or lock your joints, as both actions can lead to injury.

Conditioning: This phase should last 20-30 minutes and includes the main activity itself. You're burning calories while also experiencing the health advantages of exercise. Make a note of your intensity level (how hard you're working out) while you're exercising. As you gain strength, you will be able to devote more time to conditioning and work at a higher intensity.

Cool Down: This section should last approximately 5 minutes. This aids in the recovery of your body after the conditioning phase. Your blood pressure and heart rate will gradually return to normal. You can lower the intensity of your activity and do some of the same stretches that you did during your warm-up during this phase. Do not sit or lie down without first cooling down, or you might feel dizzy or experience fluttering in your chest.

Aerobic Exercises

Aerobic exercise promotes circulation, which lowers blood pressure and heart rate. Especially light intensity activity or light aerobic exercises work wonders to reduce blood pressure.[3] It helps your heart utilize oxygen more efficiently by enhancing blood flow. It also enhances your cardiac output and improves your total aerobic fitness, as evaluated by a treadmill test. This test evaluates how well your heart pumps. Aerobic exercise also lowers the risk of type 2 diabetes and supports blood glucose control in people who already have the disease. We suggest you engage in any of the following exercises for at least 30 minutes a day and at least 5 days a week.

Jogging and Running

Jogging, running, and biking are fun exercises as you get to pick the time and place for these activities. If you do it in a group, the experience gets even better. However, your ability to run and jog will be determined by your overall physical condition. Consult with your doctor before starting these exercises. Running and jogging are simple aerobic exercises that have been shown to improve cardiac health. Here are some tips to get you started:

- It is recommended that you walk for 20-30 minutes five days a week.

- Start with 5-10 minutes every day at a gentle tempo and gradually increase the time and speed as you gain strength.

- You should be able to converse and walk at the same time.

- If you're out of breath, take a break for 1-3 minutes and then resume walking at a slower pace.

- If your legs become weak and fatigued while walking, take a break for 1-3 minutes and then resume walking at a slower pace for a shorter period of time.

Swimming

Swimming is another low-impact way to maintain heart health. Swimming can help you achieve a variety of goals, including heart health, weight loss, pain management, and arthritis management. This is because exercising in water reduces the impact of your body weight on your joints. You don't have to wait long to reap the benefits of swimming because, in a short while, those who swim consistently can experience benefits in 4:

- amount of blood pumped out of the heart per minute
- optimal utilization of the oxygen your heart takes in from the air
- reduced heart rate
- improved Blood Pressure
- improved breathing
- refined circulation

There are two other ways you can engage in water exercises to improve your heart condition.

1. **Water Walking:** Walk across a pool in water up to your waist, swinging your arms and keeping your back straight. You can add weights after your

strength and endurance improve. Alternatively, when you become more comfortable, you can proceed into deeper water.

2. **Water Aerobics:** As your tolerance for water exercise grows, you can consider enrolling in a water aerobics class at your local gym or health center. The friendship that many people feel in a class setting is one of the advantages of taking a class.

Strength Training

Resistance training has a more targeted influence on body composition. It can assist patients with losing weight and building lean muscle mass. This is especially true of stubborn belly fat (which is a risk factor for heart disease). According to research, combining aerobic exercise with resistance training can help boost HDL (good) cholesterol while lowering LDL (bad) cholesterol. The following are some of the advantages of weight training:

- Improved Muscle Strength
- Improved Bone Density
- Greater lean muscle mass
- Loss of Fat
- Improved Insulin sensitivity
- Enhanced endurance

Resistance training is not something you should do every day. Engaging in strength training exercises on two non-consecutive days per week does the trick. Examples of strength training include using free weights (dumbbells or barbells) weight machines, resistance bands, or body-resistance exercises (pushup, squats, and chin-ups). Since hitting the gym and lifting weights requires a lot of energy, it is advisable to skip resistance training activities if you have been diagnosed with any of the following:

- unsteady coronary heart disease, i.e., angina
- heart failure
- serious pulmonary hypertension
- aortic stenosis with severe symptoms
- acute heart infection
- uncontrolled high blood pressure
- Marfan Syndrome
- aortic Dissection

Since resistance training exercises have been mentioned in the earlier chapters, here are some useful tips for strength training beginners:

1. Begin by setting an easy target. Try doing a single set twice a week.

2. Lift weights at a moderate-to-slow regulated speed in a systematic manner.

3. Lift the object through a complete range of motion.

4. Exhale during the contraction phase and inhale during the relaxation phase of the lift instead of holding or straining your breath.

5. Lifts for the upper and lower body should be rotated.

6. Weight training for healthy adults should begin with 8 to 12 repetitions each set. Use significantly lighter weights and do 10-15 repetitions each set for older individuals.

7. Chest press, shoulder press, triceps extension, biceps curl, pull-down, lower-back extension, abdominal crunch/curl-up, leg press, leg curl, and calf raises are all good exercises to undertake.

Flexibility

Flexibility workouts aim to extend the muscles' ranges of motion through slow movements. Stretching, Tai Chi, and yoga are examples of flexibility exercises. They are also used to minimize injury and strain before and after exercise. Benefits of these exercises include:

- improved balance
- better range of motion
- less painful joint movement

FAQs About Exercises After a Heart Attack or Surgery

1. How do I get back into shape after a heart attack?

Even if it's only for two minutes, gentle walking is the best approach to start. Do the best you can. Do it every day until it becomes easy, then gradually increase the time and tempo. By weeks four to six, you should be able to exercise for 15–20 minutes at a time.

2. Which forms of exercise are the most helpful?

Walking is completely free. You may do it at your own pace, and it can help you get in shape. After that, you can pick any activity you want as long as you doctor agrees.

3. Can't I just continue cycling, tennis, or football instead of these exercises?

We propose that you wait a few weeks until you've started cardiac rehabilitation and can be evaluated by an expert. If you had rapid treatment after a heart attack you may physically feel better quickly and want to resume your normal activities but it is still important to give your heart time to recuperate. We wouldn't encourage participating in any sport without first consulting a specialist.

4. Because of my arthritis and balance issues, I am unable to walk. What options do I have?

Swimming or aqua aerobics can be quite beneficial for people who can't walk very far. It has a low weight-bearing requirement and does not place a lot of strain on the joints. However, consult with your specialist first.

You might be eager to start your fitness regiment, but there are some signs you need to watch out for—lest you harm yourself. It's normal to be a little out of breath after exercising, but not so out of breath that you can't communicate or operate. If you experience chest tightness, dizziness, palpitations, or shortness of breath, stop and take a break. Keep track of any symptoms you experience (including what you were doing and when they occurred) and report them to your healthcare professional.

Reminders for Effective Exercise Sessions:

- Wait at least 90 minutes after a meal before engaging in aerobic activity.
- Do not skip warm-up and cool-down as they are crucial phases.
- Maintain a healthy balance of movement and sitting activities.
- When you feel dehydrated, remember to drink water.
- During the workout, take breaks as needed. It's better not to lie down after working out because it lowers your tolerance.
- Increase your exercise level gradually, especially if you haven't been exercising regularly.
- Maintain a steady pace while exercising.
- If you're unwell or have a fever, don't exercise.
- Allow a few days for any wounds to heal.
- If you have any questions about when you can resume your normal routine, speak with your doctor or nurse.

- Enjoy your exercise sessions! Pick an activity that you enjoy. Having fun makes it easier to keep to your schedule.

- Choose a range of activities, so you don't grow bored with what you're doing.

- Wear proper attire and footwear for your activity and the weather.

- Exercise should be a regular element of your routine. Make a plan to exercise every day at the same time and stick to it.

- Purchasing expensive equipment or subscriptions should be postponed until you know you will utilize them. It is possible to have an effective workout program that is also inexpensive.

- To stay motivated and on track, you might want to exercise with a friend.

References:

1. Bocalini, D. S., Santos, L. D., & Serra, A. J. (2008). Physical exercise improves the functional capacity and quality of life in patients with heart failure. *Clinics*, 63(4), 437-442.

2. Elward, K., & Larson, E. B. (1992). Benefits of exercise for older adults: a review of existing evidence and current recommendations for the general population. *Clinics in geriatric medicine*, 8(1), 35-50.

3. Young, D. R., Appel, L. J., Jee, S., & Miller III, E. R. (1999). The effects of aerobic exercise and T'ai Chi on blood pressure in older people: results of a randomized trial. Journal of the American geriatrics society, 47(3 277-284.

Chapter 12: Making Exercise a Habit, not a Chore

Now that you have a good understanding of the benefits of exercise, what exercises to do, and how to do them, it's time to bring it all together. All this information is no good if you don't put it to use—it's time to make sure exercise is part of your daily routine.

Sadly, that's easier said than done. How many days have you skipped going to the gym or going for a run because you had back pain, the very thing you are trying to get rid of? People have a plethora of excuses ready to avoid exercising. While trying to get my friends and community members to exercise, I have had to listen to a hundred different excuses myself! Some Days it's "headaches." Some days it's "too cold out!" You won't believe how hard it is to stick to a workout routine.

The trick to successful exercising is to make it enjoyable and not feel like a chore. There is no way you will do something every day if you don't like it. Start by making it easier for you. The first step is determining what time is realistic for you, how much you can devote to exercise each day. Will you try and do all your workout at once, or do you want to break it into smaller chunks throughout the day?

Once you have decided on the time you need to set every day, you can begin to find room in your daily routine. Remember that even 2- 3 sessions of 10 minutes of running or fast walking each day can provide health benefits. Look for parts of your day that are consistent. Do you eat breakfast at the same time most days? Maybe you can do a 10-minute workout before breakfast or go for a brief walk afterward. Don't rush, be steady. You do not want to injure yourself on the very first day! You may want to start with enthusiasm and energy, but you need to follow at a slow pace. It is important to understand the limitations of our own bodies. If you try to do a full-body workout the first day, even in the first week, your muscles will be sore, you probably won't be able to get out of bed for a few days, and your exercising habit-building will end.

The key is to make a plan that's realistic for you and not too difficult for your existing schedule. People struggle with making exercise a part of their life because they get overly ambitious and try to totally change their routines. There are additional ways you can incorporate exercise into your daily routine and enjoy the health benefits outside of your daily workouts. Here are some ideas worth trying:

- Take the stairs instead of the elevator.
- Work in the garden.
- Play with your grandchildren.
- Park farther away from your destination.
- Walk or bike places instead of driving, when possible.
- Go for a hike or bike ride.
- Dance to music.
- Walk laps in the mall.
- Try yoga.

Building a Balanced Exercise Plan

No single type of exercise will take care of all your fitness needs, and a well-balanced exercise plan targets aerobic health, strength training, balance, and flexibility. Now that you know how to perform exercises that promote each of these, it's time to put everything together.

The US Department of Health and Human Services recommends the following types of exercise:

1. 150 minutes of moderate aerobic exercises per week, or 75 minutes of vigorous aerobic activity (activities that are intense enough that you can't hold a conversation while doing them)

2. two or more strength training sessions per week, with at least 48 hours in between for recovery (or work different muscle groups on different days)

3. balance exercises

4. a daily stretching routine

Tips for Staying Consistent

- When on vacation, take advantage of hotel fitness centers. You can also bring along some equipment like walking shoes or resistance bands with you. You can also use the hotel pool to your benefit. Try to do some of the stretching exercises, bodyweight exercises, and core exercises outlined in this book in your hotel room if you don't have access to a gym.

- If you are caring for an ill spouse, child, or parent, it is undoubtedly taking up your time. Do a brief workout when your spouse is napping. You can also ask a friend or family member to come over so you can go for a walk.

- If your exercise partner moves away, do not be disheartened or skip exercising even for a day. Ask another friend to join you on daily walks or join an exercise class at your local community center. If you find no one, listen to the radio while walking.

- If you have moved to a new community, take it upon yourself to explore the neighborhood while out for a morning walk. Seek out activities that match your interests and abilities.

- If you are ill for a few weeks, wait until you feel better, then start your activity again. You will feel weak at first, but gradually, you can build up to your previous level of activity. Even if you're recovering from injury or surgery, you can do some activities. Talk with your doctor about specific exercises and activities you can do. Start slowly and build up to your previous level of activity.

The final thing that will help keep you motivated and active is your mindset—more specifically, your "why." We tend to wait until we feel motivated to do things like exercise, which we may not particularly look forward to. Unfortunately, motivation is fleeting and hard to pin down. It is often strongest during the planning phase, when we are most aware of our future goal.

Take some time to think about your "why." You want to be more physically fit, but what is motivating you? Maybe you want to be able to play with your grandchildren, travel, or just go for a walk around the neighborhood independently. Whatever it is, focus on that when you're feeling unmotivated. Write it down and visualize the outcome that you're working toward

1. How do you want to feel?

2. Are you doing this for yourself?

3. What is stopping you?

4. What is your end goal?

5. How will it feel once you achieve that goal?

6. Why shouldn't you achieve your goal?

In many cases, we are already aware of the answers to the above questions. The only thing that's stopping us is our own previous experiences. We have seen ourselves give up in the past, maybe more than once. We have seen it firsthand that when we encounter the tiniest problems while exercising, we give up the whole operation. Unconsciously, your mind has set its level of expectations based on those events. Now, even you don't believe in yourself. If you don't believe you can do it, you won't. So, stop judging yourself! You are not defined by your past actions. It doesn't matter how many times you have given up on exercising. What matters is that this time you will get it right!

Conclusion

"Don't let the Old Man, or Woman, in!"
Clint Eastwood

60 years is not a long time if you think about it, but it feels like ages because of the toll the years have taken on our bodies. Naturally, it becomes harder to move about and live your daily life independently when your muscles start protesting each time you move. Most people would suggest that you accept it. I however, will tell you to get your gym clothes. There is no reason to feel old and unfit when you are just 60! There is a whole life ahead of you, waiting to be lived. The weakness, stiffness, and pains you are feeling are the results of years of inactivity and unhealthy choices. Yet, they are not a permanent condition you must live with for the rest of your life. If you can easily reverse most of these by exercising and eating right. Then, why shouldn't you?

This book is my way of helping you regain control of your life. Happiness starts with health, freedom of movement, and self-dependency. That is all I want for you. I hope you have had fun reading this book. Even more so, I hope that this book helped you gain mobility and balance. While you are practicing the exercises mentioned here, I highly recommend taking your time. Do not rush through the movements or be frustrated with yourself when you see no improvement. Improvement will take time, but it will be long-lasting. You just need to be patient and remember:

The only bad workout is the one that didn't happen!

Dear Reader,

I hope that you have enjoyed my book. More importantly, I hope that you will start to build some or all of the exercises into your daily life. I cannot stress the difference it's made to mine.

Could I ask you a favor in return please? I am a new author and it's always a struggle to get yourself established. Leaving me a positive review on Amazon would help me so much to achive this. Just scan the QR code below with the camera on your mobile device and it will take you straight to the place on Amazon to do this and will only take a few minutes. I would be so grateful.

Thank you

Michael

Printed in Great Britain
by Amazon

30306766R00104